Extreme Sexuality in Women

OTHER BOOKS BY THE AUTHOR

Extreme Sexuality in Women

The Joy of Hyper-Sex

G. D. MASTERS

To order additional copies of this book, contact:
Xlibris
1-888-795-4274
www.Xlibris.com
Orders@Xlibris.com
604865

Contents

DISCLAIMER

The aim of this book is educational. It contains ideas and opinions of the author intended to be helpful, and informative on the topics addressed. Before applying any of the suggestions in this book or drawing inferences from it, the reader should first consult a health or medical care professional. Seeking professional help opens up wider worlds including this book.

The author disclaims all responsibility or any liability for loss, or risk, personal or otherwise, which is incurred as a consequence, directly or indirectly, of use and application of any contents of this book. The author is not liable for distress that could be associated with, or a consequence of reading this book. It is sold or made available with the understanding it is not intended nor does it constitute any form of medical, health, counseling, advice, therapy, or any other kind of professional services.

This book contains some explicitly sexual narrative. Discretion by the reader is advised. It does not contain any violence, thank you.

The primary function of a university is to discover and disseminate knowledge by means of research and teaching. To fulfill this function a free interchange of ideas is necessary not only within its walls but with the world beyond as well. It follows that the university must do everything possible to ensure within it the fullest degree of intellectual freedom.

Professor Woodward, Yale Alumni Magazine
Nov- Dec. 2014

*Collective modern man is a technical genius
merged with a moral imbecile.*
Distinguished philosopher, **Robert Nozick**

ACKNOWLEDGEMENTS

Acknowledgements serve as an important review of the author's intellectual and personal debts. It gives me warmest pleasure to acknowledge: Alex Comfort, M. D. author of *Joy of Sex* for personal association, inspiration, and graciousness in presenting a lecture at my workshop in human sexuality for California Medical Society; Alfred Kinsey, Ph.D., author of *Sexual Behavior of the Human Male* for inspiration at a lecture he gave to our class at Yale School of Medicine in 1947; Sher Hite, author of *The Hite Report* for ideas and personal attention when she graciously presented a lecture at my Workshop on Human Sexuality for the American Psychiatric Association in 1985; Jane Goodall, Ph.D. pioneer in discovery of wild chimpanzee behavior for her personal graciousness and inviting me to study her wild chimpanzee group at the Gombe Reserve, Tanzania, Africa, 1972; William H. Masters, M. D. and Virginia E. Johnson, authors of *Human Sexual Response and Human Sexual Inadequacy* for inspiration and kindness in presenting a lecture to my class on Human Sexuality, and meeting with my students informally at a reception at University of California, Davis, 1978; Hugh Hefner, founder of *Playboy* for blazing paths of freedom of sexuality in our society, and for recognition of my discovery of male multiple orgasm with publication of an extensive feature article in *Playboy*, May 1977; Marilyn Monroe, world wide icon of beauty and adulation for personal association in our teen age years, and inspiration to write *Marilyn; The Psychiatric Biography, 2012;* and Alayne Yates, M. D. author of *Sex Without Shame*, first fellow in my Section of Child and Adolescent Psychiatry, University of California, Davis, School of Medicine, and later Professor of Child Psychiatry at University of Hawaii, School of Medicine, Honolulu, Hawaii, who taught me much about development of healthy child eroticism and sexual development.

I am eternally grateful to several women, names withheld in recognition of privacy whose sexual interaction with me has enabled me to discover new aspects of female sexuality and of my own heterosexual life.

My patients in medicine deserve thanks for their contributions to my research in child development and sexuality. They have rewarded, inspired, and motivated me.

I wish to extend recognition to my mentors in medicine, psychiatry, sexology, and primatology: Edith Jackson, M. D. a humble pediatrician who founded the first Rooming-in Service in America at Yale-New Haven Hospital in 1945 where I served as Rooming-in Fellow (she was personally psychoanalyzed by Sigmund Freud); Harry Harlow, Ph.D., director of Primate Laboratory, University of Wisconsin, and professor of psychology who launched my career in primate research; Sally Provence, M. D., Director of Yale Child Study Center where I was a Fellow, 1951-1953; Herbert Ripley, M. D., Chairman of Department of Psychiatry, UW, School of Medicine, Seattle; Milton H. Erickson, M D., icon in hypnosis to whom I presented my case of a psychiatric patient at UW psychiatry grand rounds, and subsequently was my guide in hypnotherapy; and Luh Ketut Suryani, M. D., Ph.D., close colleague, Professor of Psychiatry, Udayana University, School of Medicine, who guided me in published research of the Balinese people, in Bali, Indonesia, taught me her unique method of meditation, and introduced me to the Spiritual World. John Money, Ph.D. Professor of psychiatry and psychology at John Hopkins University who generously gave pornography slides for my teaching human sex sexuality to medical students and professional audiences in the 1970s when this educational technique was used for the first time. Robert N. Butler, M.D., past president of the International Longevity Center in New York, a nonprofit think tank who supported my research on the elderly.

These guiding colleagues all became part of me to honor and give to others in my personal and professional life. Dr. Suryani is one of the few alive today.

Readers who have been immensely helpful with critiques are: Frank Sommers, M.D., sexologist, psychiatrist, and clinician, Toronto, Canada; Professor Micky Diamond, Ph.D., professor of psychology, internationally honored scholar on transgender and expert researcher, and on teaching and therapy aspect of pornography, University of Hawaii, Honolulu; John Merrill, M.D. Professor of Medicine, Northwestern School of Medicine, Chicago, IL; Dorian Larsen, Psychiatric Practitioner and colleague, State Hospital North, ID; Ruth Weiss, friend, advisor, and critical reader; and Stefan Mawab, M.D. psychiatrist and colleague in clinical work.

I am grateful to Charles Darwin, M.A., F.R.S of England for being my hero and role model of a father and fine human being, and for his seminal and epical scientific discovery of evolution that has guided my personal life and scientific work.

BOOK SUMMARY

T EN CASE HISTORIES of females who fit the definition of hyper or super-sexuality are described. The term, hyper-sexuality is better replaced by normal high-level exotic sexuality. Details of the cases provide understanding of why they developed this way, and allow analysis of psychodynamics. All persons written about are in good mental and physical health.

Known facts about the sexual response cycle, particularly the phase of resolution of women is discussed, and contrasted with the data from two women's experiences. It shows a refractory period comparable to that known for males. This discovery is a new contribution to the science of sexology.

The self-told stories are explicit, but not pornographic, and not intended as erotica (definition of erotica: literature *intended* to arouse sexual desire). The writing in the optional case to read of parent-child sexual interaction (Chapter seven) does not infer recommending parent-child sexual interaction. It intends to illustrate vibrant and normal healthy sexuality.

Reader, be ready for innovative ideas that may seem like revolutionary concepts and techniques.

This book gives no medical advice. It is not a how-to book. The stories do not advocate any particular type of sexuality. It does show how it happens, and illustrates how any woman and her partner can improve their sex life to almost unbelievable heights. The focus of this book is sexual knowledge as never told before.

The case reports conform to the guidelines for case reporting in the literature as written by the American Psychiatric Association Committee on Ethics. The individuals gave permission to relate their stories for benefit of science with assurance there was no hint of personal identity–all were carefully disguised.

INTRODUCTION

THE MERRIAM-WEBSTER DICTIONARY defines hypersexual as "exhibiting unusual indulgence in sexual activity." For dozens of references in books and articles about hypersexual women, see Wikipedia via Google on the Internet.

Little is known or studied about the origin of female hyper-sexuality. It is defined here as a high degree of sexual desire and activity by child or adult. One term used for hyper-sexuality is "sexual addiction," akin to other addictions such as alcohol. The Internet describes the nature of "sexual addiction" and something about the treatment. (Wikipedia) An official psychiatric label (ICD-10) is "Excessive sexual desire." (1) Unfortunately, this term implies abnormality.

It is important to note that hyper-sexuality of the erotic child are normal conditions, and not to be confused with sexual experiences in a child that some persons assume to constitute child sexual abuse or molestation. It is common for women who as a child have experienced sexual actions by adult and for authorities to state that any child-adult/adolescent sexual experiences are "molestation" or "sexual abuse." These terms are legal designations, and such acts punishable by law. They constitute specific sexual activity with a child under the age of 16, or by an adult five years older than the child. Regardless of the terminology, it is illegal for an adult to touch any portion of a child's body with a "lewd and lascivious" intent. Even in cases where it can be proven that the minor victim was a willing participant, a sex act or improper touching is still a crime because children under 18 cannot legally consent to anything.

The incidence of hyper-sexuality is not known. Only a few case histories have been published. A study of childhood sexuality stated that a child might develop hyper-sexuality if exposed to high degree of sexual stimulation. (2) Yates advised that the child should be encouraged in sexual expression with sex play and masturbation. There are numerous case reports in the literature of early childhood traumatic sexual experiences or sexual abuse causing varyingly degrees of mental distress and disorder. (3)

Such a relationship is shown in cases of two women in Chapters 5 and 6. (4)

No published case reports of positive childhood sexual experiences have drawn the connection to later hyper-sexuality. No scientific theory has been advanced that holds that early childhood sexual experiences can be the origin of the hyper-sexuality. This paper presents the hypothesis that hyper-sexuality is determined in some instances by early childhood sexual experiences.

Research studies have shown that for women 60 years-of-age and older, compared with the premenopausal age woman, eroticism expressed in sexual desire and frequency of sexual interaction, particularly intercourse, declines significantly (5, 6). All women are less likely to have sex at older ages, regardless of marital status. (7)

Typically, younger people, especially children, do not expect the parents or any older woman to either desire or be sexual. Most of the population considers such sexual behavior inappropriate. Unlike younger women, those 60+ tend to no longer dress or groom hair to show sexiness. To do so is considered as inappropriate. All of this influence inhibits, reduces, or wipes out any eroticism older women may have. Exceptions to this pattern do happen, possibly more than realized from accounts in lay magazines and the scientific literature.

With regard to the male's sexual performance at 80+ year-of-age, Masters and Johnson (8) wrote that there is no reason why it cannot continue satisfactorily into the 90s. They did not predict the possible course of sexual function in women past 70.

The first report (Chapter one) details the course of increasing sexual function and orgasm satisfaction in a woman 80 years-of-age. It contradicts the stereotype. She enhanced her sexuality to a nearly unbelievable extent with the help of her live-in partner, George, age 83. With his encouragement and teaching, she progressed to an astonishing level in learning and experience. She became hotter than the summer sun in Hawaii.

The stages of sexual development occurred over a three-month period in 2014. Data were obtained by personal interview of Jewel, and from first hand report of George's sexual experiences with her.

Her physical development, personality growth, and sexual history from adolescence to current age are detailed. This provides a perspective on her progression in social and sexual relationships over the past 65 years. It shows the ways her earlier and later life experiences contrasted with and contributed to her current state of heightened sexual function and satisfaction. She became highly erotic and super-sexual.

Discussion of known facts about the sexual response cycle, particularly the phase of resolution is cited, and contrasted with the data from Jewel's experience. It shows a refractory period comparable to that known for males.

The conclusion indicates new contributions to the science of sexology.

The personal case reports conform to the guidelines for case reporting by the American Psychiatric Association Committee on Ethics. The individuals gave permission to relate their stories for benefit of science were assured their identities were carefully disguised.

References

1. *ICD-10, International Classification of Diseases*, 1990. World Health Organization (WHO)
2. Yates, A. 1976, *Sex Without Shame; Encouraging the Child's Early Sexual Development*. New York: Wm. Morrow and Co.
3. Elliott, M. 1993. *Female Sexual Abuse of Children*, London: Longman Group
4. Hollander, X. 1972, *The Happy Hooker*, New Your: Dell Publishing
5. Karraker A, DeLamater J, and Schwartz CR, Sexual Frequency Decline From Midlife to Later Life. *J Gerentol Sci Soc Sci*, July 2011, 502-512
6. Laumann EO, Das A, Waite LJ. Sexual dysfunction among older adults: Prevalence and risk factors from a nationally representative U.S. probability sample of men and women 57-85 years of age. *Journal of Sexual Medicine*. 2008;5:2300–2311.
7. Lindau ST, Schumm LP, Laumann EO, Levinson W, O'Muircheartaigh CA, Waite LJ. A study of sexuality and health among older adults in the United States. *New England Journal of Medicine*. 2007;357:762–774.
8. Masters W and Johnson V 1966, *Human Sexual Function*, Boston: Little, Brown & Co.

PART I

TWO WOMEN, BOTH chronologically older, describe their transformation from ordinary sex life to extraordinary, even awesome sexuality. The discoveries revealed are applicable to all ages from teens to women and men chronologically older. They have a gift for everyone.

A young very attractive and highly sexual woman (Chapter 3) uses her sexual charm to seduce a colleague, and use him for greedy desires.

A Catholic nun, asexual and sexually unknowledgeable for 40 years (Chapter 4) illustrates how sexuality can quickly be awakened to the point of hyper-sexuality.

CHAPTER 1

EXTREME SEXUALITY IN AN 80 YEAR-OLD WOMAN

As AN ADOLESCENT, Jewel dated one boy for a year. She thought she was in love. Sexual activity consisted of only mild necking.

She married at age 17, felt like a child at the time. She had not had any prior sexual experience. She did not feel in love with him, and was not excited about him sexually.

Physically and behaviorally in her twenties, she was very attractive–slender and shapely body, 5' 2", weight 118 pounds, huge boobs, DD cup, relative to her body size, long wavy blond hair, and an ever ready smile. She always laughed easily, and made people laugh a lot at her jokes and clever remarks. In retrospect, she feels that she missed her calling as a stand up comedian.

Yesterday at the bank, she handed to the teller a check to cash. It happened to be for two dollars. She said, "Give it to me in big bills!" He said, "Do you think I'll give it to you in pennies?" She said, "Oh, I meant the other check [for several thousand]." Both had a good laugh.

A memorable event at work was the time she and girlfriend were manning an upscale store at a casino in Atlantic City. They went into the back room, smoked a joint, and came out laughing to tend to customers waiting to be served.

Another time, on leaving the shop, she forgot to check if the door lock was fully locked. People were walking around in the store, and no one was there to serve them, or prevent them from walking away with the store. The security guard called her boss (store owner) to report that no employee was there. She had long gone home. Her boss was understanding, and didn't fire her. She still has a good laugh about the incident.

She said that in youth, she did not realize how attractive she was. Her two sons remarked that they were proud when she came to their school because

she was "so pretty." Her photos in a Bikini at that time showed her sexiness and smashing beauty.

Out of habit, she shaves underarms. Being a natural blond, it never amounted to much anyway. She was not like Sophie Loren in her twenties when she showed a beautiful black hairy patch in armpits of which she was proud. George has a copy of the photo–pretty amazing for the most beautiful woman of the century.

Jewel has trimmed pubic bush, but never shaved it, even that along her thigh that shows at the edges of her panties and swimsuit. She has no need for a Merkin (crotch wig). She admits some people might think her showing pubic hair along thighs is obscene, but she doesn't care. Her current boyfriend admires all of it, and insists she not shave any of it. She agrees to do this. He is an admitted lover of loveliness of pretty women showing bodies from toes to head, and the more naked skin the better.

He would prefer that she not wear panties at all like Marilyn Monroe was famous for–she went NPL (no panty line). Jewel cannot bring herself to it–old fashioned. In the morning the sweet scent of pussy surrounds her body, and is detectable at a distance one foot away. He and she have a very sensitive and erotic nasal sensory system.

In early 20s, she worked at a number of jobs at high style sales shops and as receptionist in Atlantic City casinos. With her stunning figure and personality, getting jobs was very easy; she was always quickly hired–on the spot. She liked and had fun at every job she had. She accepted as natural to be hit on frequently, particularly by bosses, but always laughed it off. The idea of sexual harassment never entered her mind. Actually, she enjoyed the special attention, and laughed about it. She never accepted friendly men's come on, and offers of dates.

Sex with marriage–intercourse only--was "OK," she said complacently. Her husband never allowed her to give oral sex because he regarded it as dirty, and would not allow it. He was more interested in sex than she was. With him, she never had orgasm with intercourse.

Prior to the one-year separation with her husband in mid years of marriage, she had a five-year affair with a married man 16 years younger. Coincidentally, he had the same first name as her husband. Talking with girl friends it was often humorous because they were confused knowing which man by name she was referring to. To solve this problem, they dubbed him Clarence. They had intercourse regularly (she was on the Pill). She fell in love with him. It never occurred to her to give oral sex to him, nor did he ask for it.

Although, they met almost every day, her husband never knew of the affair– he was always at work. She managed logistics of the affair very skillfully. She never felt guilty, or like sneaking around. She did worry that her husband might find out. He never did tell him until years later when counseling advised she tell him. She was sorry that she did. Telling didn't help their relationship. Clarence

was an air conditioning installer, and completely air-conditioned her home free of charge. Her husband gave her money to pay him. Cleverly, she kept the money for her personal use.

Suddenly, her husband announced to her that he had fallen in love with another woman He abruptly left Jewel. She felt this was the greatest trauma of her life. Clarence and she continued the relationship until her husband and she came back together after being apart for one year. She was still in love with Clarence, but ended the affair shortly after husband and she went back together.

During the one-year period of separation, two cousins and a brother in law literally chased her around her apartment mauling her, and wanting to f **k her. One cousin, she had no interest in, but about the other, she felt ambivalent. She fended all of them off, and thought their sexual interest in her was laughable and "weird." She never made love with any of them. She had never been into incestuous relationships.

Her boobs, DD cup, were uncomfortable because bra straps pressed into her shoulders. Against her husband's desire and advice, she had a surgical breast reduction procedure. To dismay of all, it turned out badly. The right breast ended up with deformed shape, and lost all nipple sensation. Bummer! (This is not uncommon for this operation.) Fortunately, results on the left breast were reasonable, and retained nipple sensitivity. Bra size is now C to D. Her shape in sweater or blouse is still eye catching. Her boyfriend focuses touch on the left one, treats it right, and makes the most of it. As a boob man, he doesn't want to hear tell of the surgical damage because "no one likes to see a grown man cry."

With husband's rather sudden death from cancer five years ago, for the first time in life, she felt "free to do anything I wanted in the whole world," including with men. She blossomed, and felt exuberant like "a little kid turned loose in a candy shop." Her stunning body shape and beauty stayed with her. At many public places, she was hit on frequently. She took a number of men to bed to try them out.

Since being widowed six years ago, she has had a total of seven long-term relationship/sex partners. With the first one, she fell in love at first sight (first time in her life to fall in love at first sight). He was a very handsome single man 15 years younger. In appearance, he reminded her of Clarence, the man of her love affair years ago. They saw each other frequently, and slept over at her condo for one-year duration (he lived on a large sailboat at the harbor nearby). He was a very good lover. In this relationship, she, at 75 years-of-age, learned for the first time to suck penis, and enjoyed it.

One year into the relationship, she made a big mistake. She said to him, "I think I'm falling in love with you," and suggested they live together. It was the "kiss of death," and he slowly dropped her. Unknown to her, he had several other girlfriends at the time. They remain friends to this day, and speak occasionally.

At this time, she simultaneously had two other lovers. One was also 15 years younger than she. They met on POF like the others. This man came in town for three-month stints to work, and each time they resumed their sexual relationship as if an interval break never happened.

In these two relationships, she was a cougar–not intentionally seeking out men younger than she, but it just so happened. She never mentioned her real age to any man. Most people take her to be 20 or more years younger than her true age. In public situations when she has to say her real age, strangers always exclaim in disbelief, "No! Impossible!"

The third man who she came to date for a total of four years was eight years older.

She dated all three lovers simultaneously. All of them knew about each other, and accepted this situation. For her, this sexual pattern fits the definition of polyamory (multiple sex partners all of whom know each other and are accepting of the arrangement). She was not aware of the concept at the time. This pattern of desire for and sex with multiple sex partners simultaneously, even daily, may fit the definition of nymphomania, although she didn't feel like it. Real nymphomaniacs usually have indiscriminant sex with many men.

The third one, she kept for two years into her current relationship. She dated him, and took him to her bed once a week. Each three men knew about each other, and accepted the situation. Again, she was acting polyamorous, and still was not aware of the term. Finally, she told him it was over, the reason given she is dating exclusively. They remain friends.

She met current boyfriend on the Plenty of Fish (POF) "matching" website. She has never taken her picture and profile off of it. She gets at least four messages from men every day up to the present day, ages ranging from 20s to 70s wanting to meet her. Hundreds of men have written. She looks at the handsome ones. In the past year while George was looking for women to meet on POF, she answered several messages, and dated several of the men for coffee. Out of curiosity, she had coffee with one whose message was particularly sexually explicit. In person, she thought him weird, so never followed up his persistent e-mails to meet again. Now without hesitation, she simply does not respond to all inquires by men who want to meet her.

Changes in Jewel's sexuality when with current sexual/relationship partner

With present partner, for the first time in life, she has become multiply orgasmic, and it never fails to happen with oral sex (licking and sucking pussy and clitoris). The sequential full body orgasms happen at less than 30 second intervals. She has up to 10 orgasms in less than 10 minutes. Usually three and occasionally six orgasms from oral are all she is able to stand before getting the excruciating

feeling her mind "will explode." This feeling, she describes as "ecstasy." During these orgasms, she exhales. "Oh god. Oh god" repeatedly. Other frequent statements are, "You are so great," "You are the best lover ever," "It's better than ever," and "Suck me, suck me."

A few minutes after the orgasms from oral sex, she may take in hand the ready electric vibrator at bedside, and apply it to the clit. It can elicit up to three or four more screaming rock-the-walls orgasms. After that, she can take only one more clit sucking before pleading, "No more, no more," clasping thighs tightly together, and rolling onto her side. With orgasm and afterglow, her thigh muscles twitch rapidly and rhythmically.

For a single lovemaking session, a total of 12 orgasms are her maximum. Average number of orgasms per day is 16; number of orgasms per week is 100 or more.

In relationships prior to her current one, her frequency of orgasms was two or three times per week, each with intercourse. With all previous sex partners, her orgasms were usually limited to one in any single session of intercourse. None of these orgasms with intercourse had the powerful exotic character of the orgasms she has come to experience now with oral sex.

She finds that smoking pot just before lovemaking increases sexual desire and orgasms by about five fold. She is crazy about this side effect. Other women have talked about experiencing this phenomenon. Her former lover, Clarence was the one who introduced her to marijuana, and she never regrets it.

She often moans regretfully about how she has lost 60 years of good sex life—"what she could have done, and what she should have done." She said that she would make up for it now, and hopefully continuing till age 100.

While getting oral sex from George, she has the physiological reactions of swollen labia, swollen breasts and stuffy nose. It has long been known that engorged labia and breasts occur along with orgasms. Her nose reactions happen simply from excitement of sexually stimulating partner by fondling without herself having orgasm. This phenomenon has not been reported in sexology literature.

Regarding sexual foreplay. Dr. Ruth, sex expert on TV series, stated, "Just as a sexual episode does not begin with orgasm—it *requires foreplay* leading up to climax." This generally consists of talking, showing the body sexily, kissing, fondling, caressing, etc. This is a very important concept for all lovers to know and practice in order to have successful and highly satisfying lovemaking. All sexologists agree with this in general.

However, in Jewel's case, such is true only some of the times making love. When she dresses sexy, she says, "I feel sexy." However, when they awaken in bed at two to five A.M. expecting to have sex, they may neither need nor have foreplay. She may silently present herself by spreading legs, or he may move them apart. Nonverbal signals are usually sufficient. He may whisper simply, "ready for

sex?" Or, "I want to lick you." No verbal response is needed. She has told him, "don't ask–just to do it."

With her husband, she never spoke up about what she wanted. With her present partner, she feels free to speak while having oral sex. With high excitement and orgasm, she commonly exclaims like, "Oh God, oh God, oh God" "Oh my God!" "No one does it like you!" "You are the greatest!" "Suck, suck it!" "You are sooo good to me." "Take me–anything." "You can have everything you want." "I want it, I need it." "You are so good!" These words are not lost on him.

He may whisper, "I want to make you feel good." She may respond, "You do, daddy." Once during afterglow, she said, "You are my sex toy–I mean my sex boy--my sex boy toy!" The slips of the tongue gave both hearty laughs. She commented how her legs are weak. In answer to his question, "How do they feel?" she said, "Scrambled legs." "This was the first word that came to me," she said, and laughed.

She feels oral sex alone is enough to reach the pinnacle sexual satisfaction. His saliva spit on clit makes pussy and clit wet enough so personal lubricant is not needed.

Along with oral sex orgasms, he occasionally finger fucks her vagina. This adds excitement. On occasion, she has learned to enjoy his finger in anus. The anal ring is tight, and relaxes with penetration. This is not consistently a desire.

Pussy smell always revolted her in lifetime. She felt her pussy was "dirty."

George helped her reframe her attitude to feeling positive about it–a delicate fragrant odor. Now, she has come to enjoy the smell of pussy on her hand from caressing the area, as does her partner. She follows George's requests, not to wash pussy with soap so as not to disguise or destroy the natural pussy smell. It's a turn on for him. He may spend minutes inhaling down there. He has said, "I could die here [nose in pussy]--let me."

She has come to recognize the multiple body-mind sensations following final orgasm are parts of the total orgasm experience.

Satisfying post final orgasm body-mind sensations and experiences include: a) tingling sensations throughout entire body from toes to head; this, she finds particularly exotic, and wishes it would never go away; b) sensing "vibrations" in her pussy and pelvis; c) awareness of swelling and hardening of breasts; d) stuffiness of nose to point of inability to breathe through it.; e) wonderful indescribable feeling in her pussy, or as if whole body is pussy; f) feeling her whole body is pussy, and her body melts into her; g) her whole body vibrates; h) desires partner to take a handful of pussy in his hand to hold for as long as possible, up to 45 minutes;) feelings that the clit wants to be touched, and leads her to caress it, a feeling that is different from masturbation, and does not lead to orgasm; i) desire for partner to hold her swollen breast and or pussy in his hand for as long as possible. Touching her body anywhere feels "wonderful." j) orgasms that enable her to forget and ignore a persistently painful left shoulder.

The pain returns following all of the above sensations; k) feels impelled to tell her partner that she loves him, and that he is the most fantastic lover she has ever had; l) desire and pleasure in hearing her partner saying or whispering repeatedly in passionate voice that he loves her; m) verbalizes all sorts of sex talk. Says, "You have mad a monster, Doctor Frankenstein! (Wording of the Mel Brooks' movie, *Young Frankenstein.*) And I love it. Keep it up!" "Like God, you made me! You're a SEX God."; n) After orgasms likes to feel and hear the sound of his hand spanking her pussy for about 10 swift swats occasionally. This mild S & M is new for them. Occasionally, he spanks her bare butt to tease if she has been a "bad" girl. She interprets it as for being a good girl, and enjoys it; o) feelings of calm, peace and relaxation; and m) fells like she is floating; n) anticipation of more lovemaking sessions.

These body-mind sensations and feelings post orgasm last 45 minutes or longer. During this time, they fill her body-mind without conscious control. The pleasurable full body tingling sensations gradually fade over about 10 to 20 minutes time, and then cease, only to return after the next orgasmic session, and they always do. When he asks, "Did I do right?" She moans, "Everything you do is right." Moaning lasts up to 30 minutes.

All the while post orgasms, she desires to be held tightly. His firm grasp conveys a feeling of deep love filling her body/mind, a feeling she loves and cherishes. Twitches of thighs and pussy continue for up to 30 minutes. She says that these are feelings of body pleasure–feeling wonderful. She prefers that he continue to hold her whole body and/or her pussy and breast as long as he is comfortable. This adds to her continuing whole body pleasure. She says ecstatically, "Everything feels good. When he holds onto my pubic hair and pulls on it, I feel like the Stone Age women who like to be pulled by their head of hair by cave men."

Dr. Ruth, sex expert on TV series wrote, "Sex should not end abruptly. The period that follows orgasm is called the afterglow, or technically resolution–the final phase of the sexual response cycle. Both partners feel relaxed and it is a good time to share feelings and emotions." However, neither Dr. Ruth nor any other sex experts have described the feelings and emotions of afterglow (resolution) as are outlined above. This is a contribution to sexology literature.

Post-orgasms, she and George enjoy and are enlightened to discuss feelings of their lovemaking session. Initially, she felt "greedy" about wanting and having so much sexual satisfaction, much more than she felt she gave to him. He helped her reframe that feeling to a positive attitude of acceptance. She changed the feeling of greediness to shouting, "I love it. I love it." Talking about all feelings gives her satisfaction of always learning more about her mind and body.

She says happily that he created a "monster," and a "sex maniac." "I'm crazy about sex, and don't pretend to be anything else." "Knowing who you are is confidence." She actually likes these terms and phrases applied to her. In sexology

terms, she is called hypersexual, hyper-erotic, or super-erotic. When he mentions to her that she has become a changed into to a highly sexual woman, she smiles in satisfaction, and always says, "*You* made me this way."

When dressed up in sexy lingerie to show off, she points proudly to the pussy hair that comes out of her gown and shows along side her thighs. She never shaves it any more. She buys more alluring clothes to wear in public, and gets compliments from strangers. She buys lingerie including thigh high black fish net stockings to wear with high heels to display seductively in the evening at home. No longer does she compulsively wear panties to bed, and usually goes completely naked. She says she thinks sex all day. She frequently picks up her sarong to flash naked boobs or pussy with a sultry smile. These behaviors began recently.

She had prior experience giving and getting oral sex with men in the past five years, but never before had she experienced the feelings from lovemaking as with her current partner. Prior to him, she had never before talked with any lover about her or his sexual feelings. She said that with her other lovers, after his or her single orgasm, they usually turn over in bed and go to sleep. This is typical for most couples.

She has also come to realize and accept that she has become "sex crazed." This means that during the entire day, she thinks about the sex more than before the learning experiences noted above. Her thoughts of sex far exceed the average frequency of the female, two to three times a day. During the day thoughts may spring into her mind of him sucking her clitoris, each time sending a surge or heat throughout her body. Now, she wants active sex repeatedly each day–at least two, and sometimes three times. Daily sex sessions may occupy as much as six or more hours in total. They seldom miss a day of sex (e.g. as happens when on extended air flights to Europe, or when traveling alone to visit girlfriends on the East coast). Fortunately, as retired, they have the time for the frequent lovemaking.

She has become inspired to show herself dressed sexually, and act sultry for her partner. She feels more romantic, and likes close dancing. In behavior at home, she shows feelings of affection and attraction to George. In social situations, she is appropriately restrained. Strangers seeing them often ask if they are on honeymoon. They must be emitting images of romance.

She does not feel that she could possibly feel more sexually expressive and excited, but frequently says after each session, "It's better," or "the best ever." During lovemaking, she exclaims repeatedly, "You are the best lover in the world." "I have had orgasm my whole life, but never before like this!" Prior lovers had not inspired her to talk while having sex.

She remarked, "I think the reason you are such a good lover for me is because you like to do it so much."

Never before did she know that she had such sexual potential in her body-mind. She hopes it continues to get better, if that is possible. Lol. She can't imagine how it could ever be better.

Like most women, she had never seen her clit, or knew what it looked like.

George showed it to her in a mirror, and on an I-pad photo. It is unusually large: about a quarter inch thick, and almost an inch long when erect with stimulation, and is pulled out to full length. She was astounded at the revelation, and a bit proud. He felt accomplished by the demonstration. The clit becomes erect when licked, and the tip shines even in dim light. This makes it easier for him to locate it in the dark to suck.

She says, "My entire world has changed." She attributes the change to her partner who taught her to awaken her sexuality--feelings she had not known she had. She is ever grateful to him, and hopes he will never stop giving sex and love to her, and will stay with her to eternity. She likes him to give reassurance.

She likes to please him sexually by oral sex exciting him to orgasm as often as he is capable, which is about once in 24 hours. This frequency is usual for a man of his age. Only half of the times of orgasm does he ejaculate--also normal for men over 80 years-of-age first described by Masters and Johnson. (This is a well-known fact about the older male sexual system.) She sometimes worries that she has "not done enough (orgasms)" for him. He assures her that she pleases him perfectly fine. His penis becomes turgid as result of focusing on her pleasures. She greatly enjoys (loves) giving oral sex, and has become very skillful. Often, she begins the morning with stimulating and sucking cock.

Following a session of sex, she feels like simply lying in bed to rest with each holding the other in skin-to-skin closeness. It makes her feel good to lie with each other for up to one hour when they have nothing more pressing to do. She usually starts with face-to-face position. In a few minutes, she shifts to her right side. In spoon position, he holds her left breast in one hand, and alternates holding a handful of pussy. This touching with some movement does not usually excite her sexually, but results in "good feelings" throughout her body. She has said, "You bring out a blooming flower in me." She shouts, "I feel WONDERFUL!" "I can feel it in every cell in my body!" She feels "peaceful," and "relaxed." Sometimes so much so that she can barely get up to tend to desire to pee. When holding pussy, he detects pulsations and thigh twitching. She is unaware of these body contractions. While being held in these ways, she often falls asleep, and wants to be held as she sleeps.

The following is the sequence in a typical morning lovemaking session. It begins at about 5 A.M. when both awaken. They take face-to-face position; holding for some minutes. She gives a kiss on lips. He moves her to spoon position to hold her left breast and body tightly. This is met by her pelvic thrusts. After several minutes, he rises up, and moves her body to lie flat. Head between her legs, she spreads them more. He moves mouth to her pussy, inhales the

aphrodisiac fragrance for a minute, spreads the labia to reveal the clit, puts lips to it, and begins to swish tongue around it, or put it between his lips and suck. In several seconds, she begins to moan. The first orgasm happens in about 25 seconds (he is counting). He moves head away, and allows her to experience it for 5 to 10 seconds. As she quiets some, he goes to the clit for the next orgasm. It takes less time of licking--about 15 seconds. Repeating this sequence of five or six orgasm, the final orgasm occurs after only five to ten seconds of licking. It is the strongest and loudest. She moans, "Oh God," repeatedly.

At this point, he holds her in spoon position with hand on breast, and squeezing her body tightly. She whimpers and moans with each breath exhalation. Nipples erect again.

The "delicious" tingling sensation--head to toes--is strong throughout her body.

After 15 minutes, it subsides slowly to be felt only in the toes, and finally disappears. Pelvic vibrations persist, and intermittently, her hips thrust involuntarily against his body.

She wants him to continue holding her tightly.

He glances at the bright digital clock at the end of the bed, and sees an hour has past since last orgasm. She is now snoring quietly. When he lets his grip on her body relax or loosen, she pleads, "Don't go."

Her nose is still stuffed up, and she enjoys the feeling. Finally, he moves away, slips the sheet over her, and allows her to sleep. She lies quietly for half an hour. She will not desire or be able to be sexually aroused for the next six to 12 hours. This is the refractory phase of the female sexual response cycle–a new discovery.

With stimulation, her desire never fails to resume.

This is the general pattern of lovemaking in subsequent sessions of the day.

Discussion

This single woman of older chronological age (80 years-of-age) living with a companion 83 years-of-age experienced a major transformation of sexual function during a recent three-month period in 2014. Her sexual desire and activity increased dramatically. This pattern is unlike that experienced by most women past menopause. Studies have shown that frequency of intercourse and desire in older women is generally decreased.

Before marriage at 17 years-of-age, she had not experienced or learned anything about sex. This was before sex education in schools. During marriage of 58 years, sex life with husband was mundane with one exception: of a five-year sex/love affair in her 30s with a married man. This was a double cuckold. It signified her basically adventuresome sexual personality. After becoming widowed, she had many sex partners.

Her current lover was able to teach her many new ways to make love, particularly oral sex. Although she had had more than 10 lovers in life prior to her current partner, she did not learn to give oral sex with any of them. She usually had an orgasm with each partner during intercourse.

In the past four months with present partner, her pattern of orgasms has changed remarkably. She has up to 12 orgasms in each lovemaking session, a total of 98 orgasms per week. These orgasms are multiple (several within seconds of each), and stronger than any experienced before with other lovers. She craves sex, and desires it at least two and up to four times each day. This is a high degree of sex drive. Presently, her sexual and relationship systems can be called hyper-erotic and hypersexual. A better term is normal high-level frequent sex responsiveness.

At one three-year period following death of her husband, she could be called polyamorous. This term means a person having multiple sex partners, all of who know about each other and accept it. With current relationship, she has settled for only one man, and does not want more. Hyper-sexuality and hyper-eroticism persists. She has never had a lapse in or problem of sexual desire, or eroticism, and levels have become increasingly higher. Such significant positive change in the sexual system of any older woman (60 or more years-of-age) has not been written about in case reports.

Inadequate sexual desire is a rather common affliction of many women at or past menopause. When problems of desire happen, they can be among the most difficult sexual disorder to successfully treat even by the most skilled therapists.

Andersen and Cyranowski, Department of Psychology, The Ohio State University, made an excellent review of research in the sexual response cycle including the stage of resolution. (1) This careful review did not specify the many aspects of the cycle as presented in Jewel's case.

The phase of the sexual response cycle following orgasm has traditionally been called simply, resolution. Masters and Johnson (M & J), (2) described the physiological changes of the female:

1. Clitoris descends
2. Labia return to unaroused [their term] position and color

The Cleveland Clinic wrote few words about resolution: "This phase is marked by a general sense of well-being, enhanced intimacy and, often, fatigue."

M & J found there during resolution, there is a subsidence of all the physiologic changes of orgasm in males and females as they return to their normal basal state. Heart rate, blood pressure, and respiration return to normal. Muscles in a state of contraction during orgasm become very relaxed. Some women described their bodies as "limp." Women may describe their relaxation post orgasm as a time of complete calm, and "feelings of closeness to the partner may be at the maximum during resolution."

Behavior of resolution/afterglow is not shown on porno films and videos.

Post orgasm, Jewel experienced body and mind senses and feelings of many different kinds. All of the new sexual feelings have increased her sexual satisfaction many fold. She has come to acknowledge that she is "sex crazy," a "sex maniac," and "craves sex." She likes to be known as such to her partner.

Most of the 25 different feelings and bodily sensations with orgasms and afterward (resolution/ afterglow) detailed in Jewel's case have not heretofore been described in lay or sexology literature. Particularly significant for her are whole body tingling sensations, stuffy nose, wonderful whole body feelings, vaginal vibrations, prolonged whimpering and moaning, feeling entire body is pussy, feeling their entire body is one, feeling like floating, and sensing love from him flowing into her whole body.

These sensations can be explained as a dissociative phenomenon. Dissociation is an alternative state of conscious. The mental process has been known for thousands of years, but described scientifically since 1830. (3). Normally, people experience it often. It is a subsystem of consciousness in which things, sensations and motor activity happen without our will. The analysis of data of Jewel is new.

The stuffy nose reaction following orgasms is caused by sexual excitement of the erectile tissue in the normal nose. This physiological reaction of the nose with orgasm is seldom recognized. It is described here for the first time.

Some porno sites on the Internet show videos of women having vigorous full body convulsive like orgasms. Possibly, these orgasms are faked--not real. Extreme/violent orgasm is not described in the sexology literature.

The duration of the afterglow/resolution phase of the sexual response cycle has never before been described in the literature. One hour, as seen in Jewel's case, is a relatively long time as a part of the cycle.

Her desire to accept sex and to become excited again does not resume until six or eight hours after orgasms--she just wants to relax. At this time, she rejects his move to sexually excite her. She just says, "Later."

The reaction resembles the physiology of the male sexual system–the refractory period when another excitement phase with erection is not possible for many minutes to hours. This can last a day or more for men 80+. Sexologists have said flatly that women do not have a refractory period. Of course, women don't have it between multiple orgasms. In females, the phenomenon of mental/ body absence of sexual desire, and inability to become excited has not heretofore been described in the literature. It can be designated the female refractory period, or phase. As such, this case represents a new sexology discovery.

Commonly, the resolution phase is called afterglow. As noted from the above statements about Jewel's behaviors post orgasm, very few of her sensations have heretofore been described. The female refractory period is described for the first time.

While this single story reveals new aspects of female sexuality, it needs to be supported by replication with further research of "cases." Readers may be inspired to make observations of their own sexual interaction with partner.

Conclusion

The example of sexual unfolding of this single woman in later years of life is shows the potential of and multitude sensations in function of the female sexual system of a woman of any age when she has the erotic desire, and is properly inspired and stimulated. It is particularly relevant to the older woman. She is not over the hill. These sensations may be possible for many women who let their eroticism prevail with a suitable sex partner--they are out there. Yes, Virginia, he is real. Let all women be so lucky.

The new data in this report is a scientific contribution.

References

1. Andersen, BL and Cyranowski, JM, Women's sexuality: Behaviors, responses, and individual differences. *Journal of Consulting and Clinical Psychology,* Vol 63(6), Dec 1995, 831-906.Dec 1995; 63(6): 831–906.
2. Masters, W.H.; Johnson, V.E. (1966). *Human Sexual Response.* Toronto; New York: Bantam Books. ISBN 0-553-20429-7. 1981 edition
3. Speigel, D. (Ed) (1994). *Dissociation, Culture, Mind and Body* Washington, D. C.; American Psychiatric Association

CHAPTER 2

THE FABULOUS FEMALE AFTERGLOW IN A 60+ WOMAN

THIS CASE HAPPENED six years before that described in the original article about Jewel and George above. Corina is a 64 year-old native of Romania was lover of the unmarried American man, George, 83 years-of-age. She was widowed four years prior to meeting him on the matching website, "Plenty of Fish." The same George of the earlier report became her first lover since her husband died. They corresponded frequently by e-mail, and exchanged explicitly sexual messages expressing intentions and desires. He traveled to her city, and she traveled to his on a number of occasions. Each time they spent up to a month together.

At first meeting, they rode in the back seat of her sister's car as she drove them from the Bucharest airport to his rented apartment. She was glowing in her short skirt. He was eager to check if her statement on e-mails that she never wearing panties was true. His hand moving all the way up her thigh discovered the answer. It found the plush hair of her bush, and to his pleasure, she liked it–an auspicious beginning.

They stayed at a hotel in Bucharest, her city of residence, and the capitol city of Romania. Immediately, they made unrestrained passionate love. Every day, they made love several sessions a day. She was highly sexual, and always had orgasms with both oral sex and intercourse.

In sex history as a child, she had a "boyfriend" for several years beginning at age 10. He was a youth 10 years older than she who lived in her neighborhood. They rendezvoused several times a week at an empty house. Kissing was the only sex they had. She could not recall any other childhood sex play, and never experienced sexual abuse.

She described orgasms and afterglow. "The feelings begin immediately at orgasm, and continue for untold minutes. There is a hypersensitivity to all of my skin. It is as if every cell is lit up, and glowing. I can feel the heat of his hand even three inches away from any part of my body. Now, his touch is like that for me only; before orgasm the touch was for both of us. I feel orgasm all over my body, and feel his cum inside me. My pussy feels very big as he is inside me, all. There is warmth and pulsation in my pelvis, like in my ovaries, and I feel like having a child. There is sensation of a nerve connection between my pussy and my breasts.

"I feel myself more beautiful, young, and my breasts feel bigger and fuller. If I get out of bed to go to the bathroom, I can see in the mirror it is real."

"I lean over him lying like an angel, and kiss him many times, as I say, 'I love you,' over and over. It's like I can't stop. When we have simultaneous orgasm, all feelings are many times stronger than with separate orgasms. I am in trance."

To George's question, she answered, "What is the trance like?"

"The trance in afterglow is different than that before the big orgasm. Before it, I feel like I am running toward something, and I am totally alone, nothing around me. In trance with afterglow, feel like I have reached it, and he is happiness with me. When I look at his profile as he lies beside me, I feel like I have known him for a long, long, long time; maybe centuries–time does not exist.

"My trance is not like my mind before orgasm. Then he puts me into trance with his flow of words. Words like, "I love you. You are my gorgeous woman, my woman, always," are very important. In my ecstasy of afterglow, he doesn't have to say anything, and I can't speak. I am mostly in myself."

"It is ecstasy and happiness all over me, like swimming in love. It surrounds me. The experience is serenity. My mind is free and full of everything good; all troubles are gone. I feel in love, and like the feeling he is in love with me. I think this could only happen when both are in love. I have never felt otherwise because I have always been in love with him."

"How long does afterglow last?" he asked. "My intense feelings can last up to several hours, or a full day. It is there if I get up and out to the kitchen to get a snack, or even leave the house to buy a loaf of bread, and then go back in my bed. One morning, my hairdresser asked, 'You look so entranced, what happened.' I smiled, and said, 'I just got laid.'

"When afterglow ends, my desire for repeated sexual action may not return for up to a day. When afterglow is short like a few hours, we have sex as often as three times a day. I never tire of it, and always want more [foreplay and intercourse] like four times in the day. On those instances when I may not want to make love physically, I feel love mentally.

"How is the big orgasm different from those following it?"

"When my orgasms continue after the big one, when I scream with excitement, the afterglow ones are different. Immediately after the big one, orgasms continue as long as he stays in me and thrusts. Without my telling,

he seems to know how to keep them going. His thrusting raises my level of excitement till I reach a plateau for about 10 seconds, and I stay there until he stops. My descending to a lower level of excitement follows this. I stay there for about 7 seconds, until he resumes thrusting, and I go up again. He says, sometimes during the period of the high level, he can feel my vagina rhythmically grasping his penis. I can sense my vagina rippling. It's like taking cum up inside me to make a baby. Of course, I can't get pregnant, but the feeling and unconscious thought is there. That doesn't happen during the big orgasm.

"These 'orgasms,' as I call them, can repeat for a period as long as maybe 10 minutes. When he pulls out there are no more orgasms, and I enter the afterglow I described. Within a few minutes, a layer of sweat covers my entire body, including my head. My hair and chest are wet, as is my shirt, almost soaked. It is more than when I have only the big O." At no other time in my life do I sweat like this.

"I am a perfectionist in everything I do–at work, play, or lovemaking. Every orgasm I have is not perfect. I want it again, and again, and again because it is not perfect. I keep repeating it because I want to approach perfection. Each time, I feel I am getting closer. If you had the perfect orgasm, you wouldn't need to repeat it?"

"How different is it when you have made love, but not had orgasm?" George asked.

She stated, "If there is no orgasm, there is no ecstasy of afterglow. Lovemaking before orgasm is desire to begin, and sexual desire to keep going, higher and higher, hoping [to reach orgasm]. Like if it occasionally happens, we make love without orgasm, my sexual desire continues all the next day. Even when I go shopping, my trance state doesn't end. It's a smaller dimension than occurs with actual lovemaking to orgasm, but it exists."

Discussion

Corina's pattern of multiple orgasm and characteristics of afterglow amplifies the numerous feelings described for Jewel in Chapter one.

It is significant that being without sexual experience for four years, this older woman's sexual system functioned excellently. This belies the belief, "If you don't use it, you lose it."

Corina's afterglow reaction has similarities and differences from that stated by Jewel. An initial major orgasm was most intense, and followed by smaller orgasms. Afterglow lasted much longer–up to a full day the day following orgasms. The post orgasm sweating response was like that classically described by Masters and Johnson, but more extensive and intense. She described feelings of orgasm as occurring throughout her entire body. Her afterglow statements, "My pussy feels very big, as he is inside me, all of him." "I feel like I have known

him for a long, long, long time; maybe centuries–time does not exist." "I have the sensation of a direct nerve connection between my breasts and pussy."

All three of reactions are explainable as a normal mental dissociation process. She correctly identified orgasm experiences as happening in a state of trance. Jewel had similar experience.

She experienced a refractory period as did Jewel, but it lasted for a longer period of time–up to as long as one day. This basic reaction confirms of the validity of the female refractory period.

The frequency of lovemaking sessions and orgasms qualifies her as hypersexual, or normal highly sexual. She never had this degree of eroticism during her marriage.

CHAPTER 3

A Scholarly Highly Sexual 45 Year Old Woman

MINNA WAS A 40 year-young colleague in a similar academic field who showed her colors of excessive sexual behavior rather soon after introducing herself at a visit to his office at the university. She came to ask him to serve as a member of her graduate committee for her Ph.D. program in child development.

She was quite attractive with long natural wavy blond hair, and a rather slinky low cut dress on a slender body 5' 8." Her manner was straight forward, and the request to help her scholastically was hard to refuse. He accepted her request on the spot.

She explained the teaching she does at another university in the city. As a part time faculty member, she taught a course in human sexuality. He wanted to know more about it. She suggested he come to her office to view the movies she used in the course.

He attended one of her lectures in an auditorium packed with 200 students. She said the course is always full. She gave an impressive lecture for all students and him. He thought she would be a good co-teacher in his course in human sexuality for medical students.

She promptly invited him for coffee in her home. That seemed to him to be auspicious. She was dressed rather seductively as usual, and served tasty Danish pastry with coffee. He studied her conversation and body movements carefully. When both were standing close to each other next to the kitchen, he made his move. He leaned to her, and gave a tender kiss on the lips. Her acceptance led to his putting tongue in mouth. Again, she emitted sex vibes as they French kissed. He didn't push the encounter further. When he left, he felt sure she would make a fantastic lover.

He invited her to his apartment, and she accepted with the enthusiasm of a lover.

In the apartment, they made love. He undressed her. Topless, she showed off her lovely D cup boobs. He was hooked. After foreplay with caressing bodies and kissing, they had intercourse. She had a loud orgasm, and he shot his wad in her wet vagina. The relationship was moving fast. She acted completely ready for anything sexual.

To shorten the story, they soon became regular lovers. She was married, had three kids, a daughter 13 and two boys younger, and her arrangement seemed perfectly natural. They met at his apartment or at her house when the kids were at school, and husband was out teaching high school. She didn't mind him knowing of her cuckolding because he had a girlfriend on the side with whom he met with frequently.

In two months, she had a new request. She would like him to help her be accepted at the medical school where he taught. He being helplessly lost in their loving, agreed to do all he could to help her get acceptance at the school. She wanted advanced standing after taking the courses of the first year as a visitor. To make the subsequent events short, the assistant dean stood in the way of acceptance in the class. Meanwhile, she passed the tests for obtaining a Ph.D.

Sexually, she had a voracious appetite—at least once a day. When riding in his car, she frequently gave him a blowjob. She liked taking lonely exits off freeways to have intercourse in the car because she couldn't wait till they got home. They had intercourse on public beaches when no people were around to see. They attended medical meetings in out of town cities, including in Europe and Asia, the perfect places to dump the lectures and have frequent sex. He was able to keep up with her sexually. At one meeting in D.C., she seduced and went to bed with a man who was chairman of the grant committee of the National Institute of Health. He saw to it that her grant request was funded. She had bought it with sex. Irresponsible, she failed to carry out execution of the study granted.

This pattern went on for two years. Sexually, she was hypersexual, always horny and filled with desire.

He learned of her cheating on him. Worst of all, she secretly seduced another faculty member in his school to help her take over his teaching of sexuality. This betrayal was too much, and prompted him to end the relationship. His anger and avoidance of her lasted for years.

Comment

This young married woman easily seduced a faculty doctor to become her lover. She was so clever and he so moon struck that she was able to use him for a number of her personal greedy desires.

She was super-sexual woman using sex to get what she wanted. She didn't care where the chips fell as long as she attained her goals. Eventually, her trickery was revealed. Although happy for two years, her partner learned a hard lesson. He could do without her, and turned to other fish in the sea for sexual adventures.

CHAPTER 4

EXTREME SEXUALITY IS AWAKENED AT AGE 40 IN A FORMER CATHOLIC NUN

Abstract

A 40 year-old, Caucasian, single, never married, mentally and physically healthy former Catholic Nun who had no sex education or previous satisfying sexual experience was desirous of having sexual experience for the first time in her life. She selected a man named Stephen who had placed an ad on the personal meeting site of Craigslist. He was in his eighty's, honest, and had extensive sexual experience. With relatively small knowledge of him via e-mail exchange, she went to his private apartment fully intent on having sex, and to give what he wanted, oral sex. Two extensive and satisfying lovemaking sessions on two successive days unleashed her incredibly powerful innate sexuality. The experiences raised deeply entrenched conflicts, guilt and shame inculcated by her religious beliefs. Subsequently, she continued to express by e-mail to him strong and explicit sexual feelings and desires. Detail in the report enabled analysis of the psychodynamics.

Introduction

This case revealed is unique in our time. It is well documented that Catholic Nuns living in monasteries or convents in Europe years ago had clandestine and often forced sexual intercourse with priests. "Many of the nuns commit fornication with the very monks who are placed in authority over them; and in the same monasteries many bring forth sons and daughters." (1) Bones of newborn infants have been found buried in grounds of the places of residence.

The article, "Sexual Abuse in the Roman Catholic Church" states that 40% of Catholic Nuns have been sexually abused [by Priests]. Of those who got pregnant, their babies were murdered. (2)

Catholicism backed by the Pope strictly forbids any sexual activity by the clergy, or fornication by Nuns, as well as the unmarried parishioners.

The matter of her religion is specified in this report because it played a dramatic role in the woman's emotions and behavior, and her mental health.

The story of this woman was not a clinical case; she was not a patient. She is a religiously devoted conservative Caucasian with a good work history, and until recently a Catholic Nun in America. She is a 40 year-old, single, never married woman who had no sex education or previous satisfying sexual experience, and was desirous of having a satisfying sexual experience for the first time in her life.

She had not taken her final vows with the Church. The vow of chastity frees a nun from the demands of an exclusive human relationship so that she can "give all her love to God." By the vow, she would promise not to marry, and not to engage in romantic behavior or sexual acts.

This is the first detailed report of sexual development of a Catholic Nun recorded in the sexology literature. The purpose is education, and to understand psychodynamics of the woman living in the sexually forbidden culture of her religion.

For sexual experimentation, she selected a man who had placed an ad on a personal mating site of Craigslist. It said specifically, he wanted for a woman who would "give her breasts and clit to suck." The idea appealed to her imagination. With relatively little knowledge of him except career, age 80+, or meeting first at a neutral place such as a coffee ship, she went straight to his private apartment fully intent on having sex, and give what he wanted.

Details of the report enabled analysis of the psychodynamics.

Method

The author reports the true story of a former Catholic nun here called Alicia, age 37. She is in good mental and physical health. Direct quotes are hers. Details of her personal life, her first two satisfying sexual encounters with her sexual partner, and the aftermath, with a man, 83 years-of-age, were obtained through direct contact and e-mails.

Results

Her entire family is devoted Catholics. She entered the nunnery at age 16. She was in the Catholic Order in an Eastern city wearing the nun habit till she left the Order at age 37. In her work at a large hospital during the past three years, everyone knew her background as a nun, and called her "Sister." She enjoyed

being called sister, loved the job, and preformed energetically and excellently at it. All staff liked her.

After a life with absolutely no sex education at either school or home, she was somehow inspired at age 40 to try "branching out to see what the world of sex is like." She had never before dated. One night, she took to her apartment a stranger met on the Internet. She related, "Without foreplay, he stuck his penis in me for about a minute, 'exploded,' and abruptly left me. I didn't orgasm. It was almost like rape, although I liked the feel of it." She said admiringly, "I had never before seen an erect penis."

She had answered an ad on the public advertising site Craigslist that said, "I want a woman who will let me suck her boobs and clit." The message struck her as interesting. In e-mails, she learned of his career in the mental health field, and sexual desires. She explained frankly her interests on e-mail. In honesty, she wrote, "This may be a deal breaker. I'm five foot seven inches tall, and weigh 265 pounds." In response to Stephen's question of bra cup size, she said, DD. Startled, yet enticed by her two physical assets, DD, he reassured her that it was her, and not her overall size that interested him. She admitted that while anticipating the encounter, she was "shaking, very nervous, and scared."

She declined to meet face to face at a neutral safe place such as a coffee shop. Instead, she came to Stephen's apartment located in a lively and good section of the city.

She parked her car at a short distance from his apartment. She walked as if shrouded because she didn't want to be seen in public appearing as if on a date with a man.

This date would be the first in her life. She was adamant that no photos would be taken. At his request, she dressed in a blouse that showed cleavage between her DD breasts.

At first sight of him even though he was more than twice her age, she didn't flinch! Entering the apartment, she looked around briefly, admired it, and liked the ambience. She spoke few words. Her mind was no doubt preoccupied with accomplishing the premeditated task at hand. No drink was necessary; she never drinks alcohol and never even tasted wine. She declined even one little sip of campaign that he had bought in anticipation of celebrating.

While sitting on the couch, Stephen calmed her by holding her hand. In two minutes, she relaxed, as she laid her head gently on his shoulder. She found that she loved him stroking her hair, and was surprised because she doesn't like her hair touched; no man had ever before touched it. She let him undress her with help to unfasten the bra.

The next two hours were spent on the bed making love. She loved all of it, had a very, wet vagina, and had dozens of orgasms, large and small. Some loud orgasms rocked the walls. This was the first time in her life she had an orgasm or

multiple orgasms. Prior to this, she didn't really know what an orgasm is. "I just knew I wanted it." She had never engaged in self-pleasuring.

Well into the sex play, she took his erect penis in her hands, and gently stroked it for minutes. The erect penis mesmerized her. At his request, she played with and sucked it. After sucking, she remarked, "I didn't much care for it." She found that she loved the long and repeated loud hard spanking of her bare shaved pussy as smooth as her body. She imagined her noise must have been heard through thick walls by neighbors. Admittedly, she loved her large breasts played with and sucked. With legs wide spread, she had multiple orgasms just from sucking pussy and clit. She screamed, "f**k me, f**k me" a dozen times as if was second nature as her body writhed and thrust—totally uninhibited. It was as if she couldn't get enough. Toes being sucked tickled, and made her laugh. She said with surprise, "I never laugh." She never said, "stop" or "no more," and liked it to continue.

Two hours into love making, suddenly as if lightening struck, her demeanor changed to grave distress. She sat up straight, bowed head, shook it in a "no" gesture, and whispered, "It's not right." She repeated the words, and could not be calmed by his saying repeatedly, "It's not wrong; it's right." She called it her "logic mind--Catholic!" From then on, she could not accept even a hug. She felt urgency to leave. At parting, she said, and emphasized with finality, "I'm sorry, and I can't see you again." She meant every word of it. Stephen's face registered shock and disbelief.

Surprise! The next day, she e-mailed how horny she was feeling, and wanted to come be with him right away again this night. She wrote passionately, and said, "I'd like to put your penis between my breasts." He accepted the invitation.

This time at the apartment, she was calm, not nervous, got naked immediately, and went swiftly to the bed. She unobtrusively placed a condom on the nightstand. They spent two hours making love with the same incredible sex for her—many multiple orgasms. She begged him to be inside her. She even took two fingers in her anus with delight and orgasm. In the fit of passion, she admitted she'd like to have a "hard cock in it."

In the course of lovemaking, she had many firsts. Open mouth kisses with sucking tongues were a first for her, and she couldn't stop. Never before had she kissed anyone. She found she had orgasm from caresses to any and all parts of her body. This included breasts kissed, breasts played with, nipples sucked, body caressed anywhere, and armpits kissed. She repeatedly asked for clitoris to be touched, and this never failed to produce orgasms. She loved the S & M of having her bare pussy spanked hard.

Again, and without warning, her "Catholic logic mind" suddenly took over like an earthquake. She stopped, quickly got up from the bed, dressed, and left, as she had done the night before. With finality, she said, "I can never see you again." Stephen believed it, and calmly walked her to her car. There was no hug or even

kiss on the cheek although it was pitch dark, and no public person was closer than 100 feet--just a perfunctory handshake.

The next morning, she e-mailed.

"The truth is that you are ever so correct in what you said about me being enslaved to sex.

"You were *right* in saying that I could be fucked three times a day and love every moment of it. I've simply got to have a hard cock in me, and get more and more orgasms.

"You were *right* in saying that I could share your bed with you and another man or woman and love every moment of it as we discussed. He would fuck me over and over as you made love to my tits, and give me your cock for my mouth. Is your girlfriend into sharing you? We could do a threesome. If she's too conservative, I am still yours--never forget it!

"You were *right* in saying that I could lie there all night and let you nurse at my breasts.

"You are right that I crave my nipples to be sucked forever.

"You are right that I want my pussy eaten so much.

"You are right that I get wet half the day and night.

"You are right that I have been transformed into a sex maniac; even a nymphomaniac!

"You were *right* in saying that I need to be taken care of!

"You were *right* in saying that you are what I have been craving! And it scares the shit out of me!!!!!!!!!!!!!!!!!

"Have you found the vibrator we talked about?

"With your blessings, I now masturbate every day, and use my vibrator. I always orgasm!

"When all is said and done, my guilt is huge . . .I do have a sexual beast in me, and feel SO ashamed of it!

"I need some time...if things were only different in my life. If I didn't have my mother to care for, if I just had myself, I could be yours. I could let you tend to my needs and take care of me. But, things are not that way.

"Thank you for absolutely wonderful two evenings! Thank you for your kindness and understanding! Please stay in touch as time allows. I just know I'll come back. I can't stay away, even though my Catholic 'logic' says, 'it's not right.' F**k it. My body knows. Didn't we? I'm sex crazy, and we both know it. You know, I'm into you for the SEX. Enough!" She enjoyed my praise of her prose.

She said honestly that she was getting ready to leave the State for two weeks, and a sweet e-mail ended expectantly, "I would like to hear from you by email if you have the time."

A day later, she sent this e-mail. "My nipples miss being sucked. I NEVER thought I'd like it SOOOO much! Playing with my boobs feels so good. You taught me, and now I'm spoiled forever! I actually like it more than my clit

sucked! I need to process your idea of being with you and another woman. I am interested in learning. :) I'll stay in touch as I can . . .Thank you for accepting me. It means the world to me. You flatter me! Thank you!"

In follow up e-mail, she wrote: "Is it possible to exchange the dildo you mentioned for a slightly smaller one that has a clit stimulator on it? Although I do not have personal experience, I have watched porno videos on my computer. When two women do each other it seems the dildo in the pussy and the vibrator on the clit make for large orgasms. And, yes, I would like to watch porno with you. I would be honored to take up your offer to visit the sex shop, and have you buy sexy things for me. You spoil me."

He answered, "The dildo I have is the right size for your vagina. I know because I had four, yes four, of my fingers in it at once, and your wet cunt took them with ease, extreme pleasure and orgasm."

In next morning e-mail, she wrote: "Good morning. Has your girlfriend returned? Is she into sharing you? I do desire a threesome. Does she shave her privates? I try to sit and dream about what it would be like to go down on her, and lick her clit until she came.

"I am getting quite the stirring thinking about being between her legs. Imagine me between her legs, and you using the dildo to fuck me from behind. I would make sure that while I licked her clit, I put my fingers in her to rub her G spot. I would stay down there until she begged me to stop. Then, I would ask her to do the same for me. I would suck on your nipples while she ate me. I would start off by touching her, then kissing her pussy, then work my way to her breasts and so on... I hope she is willing. Oh, I'm getting excited just thinking about it! I just wish I could be with you now, or even for two hours.

"I'm glad to be reassured she is clean, and for sure does not have HIV."

Two days later she wrote: "In response to your question, I don't know if I am a Nymphomaniac. I do admit to being a sex maniac–you did it, damn it! I am scared to know the truth. I wonder if my cravings are simply because I only started [sex] after 40?

"Last night, I dreamed of a 'gangbang' with a group of men! It is so vivid and colorful in my mind. We were somewhere in a private luxury room. Each man whom I could not recognize ate me, then fucked me anyway they desired–front and backside. Their playing with my big hanging tits was also sending me out of my mind. Even two men at once! While they did that, you nursed on my nipples, and I played with yours. I made you ejaculate by imitating with my mouth on your breasts what you did to me. I think I had orgasm in my sleep. I was wet. When all was said and done, we showered together. You soaped me up all over; pussy, tits, and all. So divine and erotic! Sensual! I realized this was my first shower with a man. Then, we had a private session, as I sucked your cock and massaged your prostate like I knew how until you fell asleep. Just loved that dream!"

He asked her if she thought of having a gangbang in reality? She answered quickly and succinctly: "Embarrassingly, I do!"

"It's hard to express and sometimes hard to accept this new sexual desire within me. But, my nipples do long to be sucked on at this moment!!

"It is really scary. It's like I am two completely different people. I am this sex-crazed person at night and this shy, guilt filled person during the day. OMG what is wrong with me? If I had had a more normal development or environment growing up maybe I wouldn't be sex crazed."

She wrote many e-mails asking that she could come over again, and if he could arrange a threesome with Sally, Stephen's girlfriend. He talked with Sally, and she was extremely reluctant. After long discussions, she finally relented. Alicia came to his apartment as before. With brief introductions, she slipped off her clothes. All three went to the bed.

In bed, Alicia went down on Sally who spread her legs. She liked Sally's pussy till she came. She appeared to enjoy it. Then, Alicia came to him, and invited his sucking her boobs. This produced the usual multiple orgasms in Alicia. At first, Sally watched, but soon left them to go into the living room. For about half an hour, Alicia had multiple loud orgasms. When they came out, he indicated it was time to quit. Alicia dressed, and left.

In the days following that threesome, Alicia e-mailed a number of times asking if they could do it again. Each time, he answered that Sally would not accept a repeat–no way. Although, Sally admitted that she had enjoyed Alicia's licking, she regarded it as a one-time thing. She disparaged Alicia's very overweight body, and said if it were another woman, slender and cute, it would be a different story. Alicia stayed disappointed.

They stayed in touch by brief e-mails. Alicia kept hoping for another meeting.

She wrote of masturbating while imagining him on top of her. She said that she has done it only rarely recently. "My Catholic influence," she said.

"It's hard to express and sometimes hard to accept this new sexual desire within me. But my nipples do long to be sucked on at this moment!!

Two weeks later

"Do you think your lady, Sally, will ever let me come?"

"Please let me know when she will be gone and I will try to arrange my schedule."

Stephen wrote back. "Here's the plan; I will be alone at home after 4 PM. and free for probably two days. We could have 2 days together. Isn't that WILD!!!

Tell me when you will come for our fun, loving, and sex. I will be ready 4U."

Five days later, Alicia wrote. "I have thought long and hard about this, and I need to tell you that I won't be coming any more. Although you taught me a lot, and I did enjoy our time together, I cannot justify the behavior with my moral beliefs.

I wish you and Sally nothing but the very, very best!!!!!!! With gratitude, Alicia."

Two days later, she wrote. "Dear Stephen: Thank you for your well wishes! I am torn. My sexual self wants to come, but my moral self tells me otherwise."

Two weeks later

"Do you think your lady will ever let me come?"

"Please let me know when she will be gone, and I will try to arrange my schedule."

Five days later, Alicia e-mailed.

"I have thought long and hard about this, and I need to tell you that I won't be coming any more. Although you taught me a lot, and I did enjoy our time together, I cannot justify the behavior with my moral beliefs. I wish you and your lady nothing but the very very best!!!!!!! With gratitude, Alicia

"Dear Stephen: Thank you for your well wishes! I am torn. My sexual self wants to come, but my moral self tells me otherwise.

"I am sorry, but I can't do this. My moral compass won."

Discussion

Alicia began e-mailing in polite restrained appropriate language. Following the two sexual experiences, she became surprisingly explicit in detailing her strong erotic desires and feelings. Stephen's few suggestions set off intense eroticism in her. Her dreams became graphically erotic. All this was new for her, and represented growth in freedom to express her sexuality both unconsciously (in dreams) and consciously.

It is not known why she had urge to have the first sexual experience on this particular occasion, and at this time in midlife. A possible underlying factor: was leaving the asexual sexually repressive nunnery, and release of sexual prohibition by voluntarily leaving her nun identity status with its associated sexual repression. For her to leave the Catholic Order after being a member for so many years showed basic courage and independence. Her twenty-five years of maturity as a nun from adolescence to middle age is a long time in forming mindset. Possibly, her first less than satisfactory sexual encounter a year ago could have stimulated further curiosity about sex. She was perusing the Internet site category of "Men seeking women." One caught her eye and curiosity, and she explored it by e-mail.

She was unbelievably sexually naïve: never kissed; never had any sex education or experience; never read about sex; never before spoken about sex; never heard of S & M; and had never seen sex scenes in movies or on ordinary TV channels, of which many saturate our society. She does not watch TV. Prior to the sexual experiences, she had never seen pornography. A first viewing porno on the Internet stimulated her curiosity about a dildo.

American culture is inundated with sex messages and images including the TV commercials. This day and age, it is hard to avoid it. She never thought about sex till rather suddenly self-awakened to the idea. Experiencing satisfying and extensive sex for the first time immediately opened the floodgates of sexual desire.

In terms of sexology it is significant that the female sexual system never used for 40 years can be ignited to such a fiery degree. She became hot. She speculated that it was because it began only after she was age 40, or possibly because of her "restricted life and environment [as a nun]." She wondered about possibly becoming a "Nymphomaniac," and thought she was a "sex maniac." She said, "I'm scared to know for sure."

Contrary to the sexual misadventures reported in the Catholic Church (1, 2), Alicia's introduction to sexuality in no way constituted abuse or molestation. Rather, she invited sexual action at her desire, time, place, and pace. She was fully cognizant of what she was doing voluntarily.

Typical elements of sexual abuse and molestation by the perpetrator are: initiation at a young age before the child has developed rational thinking; pressure; pursuit for the sexual pleasure of the abuser; forcing; belittling; humiliation; threats even to kill if not kept secret from any other person; deception; giving drugs or alcohol to sedate the victim in order to make the victim more pliable to exploitation, persuasion by perpetrator using religious brain washing such as, "It will bring us closer to God;" and physical and emotional abuse. None of these dastardly strikes were present in Alicia's sexual experiences.

Her last recent e-mails showed that her life had been changed forever erotically. She is very intelligent, a capable experienced medical professional, and is on a personal mission to experience sex she desires and enjoys.

She set out to explore the possibility based only on a personal ad by a horny man she had never met, and without first meeting at a neutral safe place such a coffee cafe. Going straight to his room showed courage. She was under fear of being seen by someone who might know her. Hardly any young woman would put herself at such risk of possible danger. This was the first time she had done such a thing. She must have formed good judgment via the e-mail exchanges.

How could she feel sexually free and uninhibited in a strange place with a totally strange man much older than she? It is unusual that a woman in 40s, or actually any age, would accept having a sexual encounter or relationship with a man more than twice her age. (Some movie stars are the exception. The famed movie star, Charlie Chaplin married a woman age 18 when he was 60 years-of-age.) Very few women are age blind--age not an issue. Quality and security are more important. At first sight of him, she did not show any surprise or hesitancy. Age and was not a concern for her. She did not have a "father issue." She said she was "Daddy's' little girl," and she adored him. During passionate lovemaking, she accepted his calling her "daddy's girl."

There is no hint as to why the sudden change in sexuality happened. No theory about sexuality explains it. An analysis of psychodynamics lends understanding.

There is a normal mental mechanism that allows one to shift swiftly from one attitude or mental state into another. It is called dissociation. All people do it every day in many situations. For example, when children play with a doll as if it is a real baby or have an imaginary companion, they are dissociating.

Alicia showed a sudden shift in feelings and attitude in going from total sexual abandon to feeling despair that she had in essence committed a mortal sin. Her facial expression went from ecstasy to holding head down and shaking "no," a frown, appearing as if in disaster, wet eyes, and near crying. Repeatedly, she spoke softly, "*It's not right.*" Although he tried to comfort her, and said, "It *is* right; you are good," it did not faze her. At this point, she couldn't even stand a hug. Along with it was intense guilt and shame. She did not cross her chest or say Hail Mary's.

The origin of her discomforting response was rigid Catholic upbringing. The guilt and self-recrimination was a heavy load to have been laid on her. It may never be relieved. To say of her sexual feelings at confessional would undoubtedly result in laying on more guilt with despair. Some patient's stories reveal that Priests do not understand how to manage this situation in positive healthy ways. They usually only suggest, "Don't do it again." "Pray for contrition, and do 10 Hail Mary's."

She did understand that her Catholic mindset interfered with expressing sexuality, and caused paralyzing guilt and painful shame. But, the emotions released in her body and mind over road deeply ingrained sexual inhibitions.

She may have had compulsivity that took over with sexuality once she experienced it. She did not have any other compulsions. She couldn't understand her intense desire. She had no evidence or symptoms of any personality disorder.

She came to realize what a powerfully sexy woman she is, both in desire and freedom of expression. Realize this woman had never spoke about sex before in her lifetime.

She wrote, "The truth is that you are ever so correct in what you said about me being enslaved to sex." "You were *right* in saying that you are what I have been craving!"

In terms of good mental health, her need is not to deny desire, but to accept it without shame. Counseling or therapy by an expert in the field of sexuality could help. Given her desire for complete secrecy it is unlikely she would seek or accept it.

Her immediate sexual responsiveness to the extreme is not at all typical of normal female sexuality as for example recorded and written by the ultimate experts, Masters and Johnson in *Female Sexual Response* (3). Long repressed

emotions simply exploded in her body, and would not quit until her religious based "logic" emerged to squelch it temporarily.

Her vacillation between desire to see him again, and not ever again, is betrayed in her e-mail asking about the vibrator as if she wanted to try it with him at a next meeting.

She is mentally healthy. All the while expressing her newfound sexuality, she continued to give responsible care of aged mother living in her home, needing medical attention and care 24/7. She is a dear woman.

The writer wondered if her newly emerged sexuality would be permanent, or if it would succumb again to her Catholic mindset. The answer came on 12/14. She wrote: "I have thought long and hard about this, and I need to tell you that I won't be coming any more. Although you taught me a lot, and I did enjoy our time together, I cannot justify the behavior with my moral beliefs. I wish you nothing but the very very best!!!!!!! With gratitude, Alicia."

She snaps back into sexual desire. "It's hard to express and sometimes hard to accept this new sexual desire within me. But my nipples do long to be sucked on at this moment!!

"It is really scary. It's like I am two completely different people. I am this sex-crazed person at night and this shy, guilt filled person during the day. OMG what is wrong with me? If I had had a more normal development or environment growing up maybe I wouldn't be sex crazed."

This case report conforms to the guidelines for case reporting in the literature as written by the American Psychiatric Association Committee on Ethics. The individual gave permission to relate her story for benefit of science with assurance there was no hint of her identity-- it was carefully disguised.

Summary and conclusion

This unique report in sexology literature is of a 40 year-old, single, never married former Catholic Nun who had no sex education or previous satisfying sexual experience, and was desirous of having sexual experiences for the first time in her life.

She selected a man who had placed an ad on a personal mating site. It said specifically, he wanted for a woman who would "give her breasts and clit to suck." The idea appealed to her imagination. With relatively little knowledge of the man, or meeting first, she went straight to his private apartment fully intent on having sex, and to give what he wanted.

It proved to unleash her incredibly powerful normal innate sexuality, along with deeply entrenched conflicts, guilt and shame inculcated by her Catholic religious beliefs. Although she said after first meeting that it could never happen again, she contacted him the next two months expressing desire for repeat sexual

experiences. She expressed sexual desires by e-mail until a final change of heart based on her moral beliefs.

Detail of the report enabled analysis of the psychodynamics. The report has scientific merit for the literature on sexology.

References

1. "What Goes on in Nunneries," Google search, (2014)
2. "40% of Catholic Nuns have been sexually abused." Darryl Eberhart, Editor of ETI & TTT (on Internet)
3. Masters, W.H. & Johnson, V.E. (1966) *Female Sexual Response*. Boston: Little Brown & Co.

PART II

AMAZINGLY HIGHLY SEXUAL
WOMEN OF HISTORY

Six WOMEN, TWO living today and four from collected history, illustrate the condition of what can be called super-sexuality, hyper-sexuality, or just plain normal extreme sexuality. One woman is the iconic Marilyn Monroe. All the women are normal mentally. They glory in the joy of sexual expression.

CHAPTER 5

AMAZINGLY HIGHLY SEXUAL WOMEN OF HISTORY

Two EXTREMELY SEXUAL women have written autobiographies or memoirs that contain data relevant to the origin of their patterns of sexuality throughout life.

Catherine Millet, a professional art critic and writer living in Paris in the latter part of the 2000s wrote a biography of her sexual life. Reviewers stated it was the most explicit book about sex ever written by a woman. At age 18 when she first ran away from home, she joined up with several young men who encouraged her to have group sex for the first time in the weeks following deflowering. She followed by having sex with innumerable anonymous men at orgies in Paris–up to 40 or more in a night. She realized this was unusual in the milieu in which she was brought up. She had no preferences and accepted any and all men who came in droves in all sorts of private and public venues such as city parks, day or night. Additionally, she had sex regularly with several steady partners, their friends, and associates connected with her work in two, three, and foursomes. She had sex occasionally with women, but did not particularly prefer it, and did not regard herself a lesbian. She did not use the word, bisexual, but it would be appropriate for her sexual orientation. Although she had occasional fantasies of being a high-class prostitute, she was awkward at accepting money for sex, and never asked for any money. She preferred oral sex to "fucking,' felt she had a gift for it, and was a consummate performer as she describes explicitly. Her giving oral sex was in higher in quantity than was intercourse. It is a wonder that she was infected with STD (the "clap" or gonorrhea) only twice and never became pregnant. She had a longstanding male relationship, but never married. Her pattern of sex continued throughout her lifetime. She was highly successful in

her field, very intelligent, and in no way could be considered a mentally deranged person. She did not abuse alcohol or drugs.

Her book, *The Sexual Life of Catherine M.* (2001) is astounding in content though not pornography, and one wonders how such a person and personality came to be. Was it childhood experiences, family influence, environmental circumstances, culture, hormonal imbalance, genetics, or psychology? Could it be a combination of these possible factors? The answers are provided in this article that focuses on the psychodynamics.

Data from Millet's book is sufficient for definitive analysis.

Childhood experiences. Beginning in earliest age, three and four, she had an obsession with numbers. She daydreamed about how many husbands she could have at once or in succession—six or more, or many more, even countless husbands. She wondered how she could go about it when she grew up. When married, "how many children could I have, was six the most acceptable or could I have more? What sort of age gap should there be between them, and what would be the ratio of boys to girls?"

As a child, she had established "a relationship with God" which meant every evening she had to think about what he would eat, fussing over the size of helpings, the rate at which they were served, etc. "I was very religious, and it could well be that my confused perception of the identities of God and his son favored my inclination to counting." When old enough to go to Sunday school, she told the priest she wanted to become a nun, and wanted to have multiple husbands and children. He brushed her off.

At times when she had multiple sexual contacts, she thought of the numbers. She was the one who initiated the orgies—"something I still cannot explain to myself." "I always thought that circumstances just happened to mean that I met men who liked to make love in groups or liked to watch their partners making love with other men. The only reaction I had (being naturally open to new experiences and seeing no moral obstacle) was to adapt willingly to their ways." She did not "make a theory" of this.

Childhood sexual play at age seven had a seminal effect on her perception of desire to have anal sex or rear entry that she preferred. "I had a predilection for sensations in my rump." At age six or seven, she exposed her ass to her brother in a game that included some moves she made to masturbate. She would crease her panties up into the front of her crack, and would push her buttocks out as far as she could beyond the back of the bench she was sitting on. She would then pretend to have revealed herself absent-mindedly, and he pretended to brush her bare buttocks inadvertently.

In this play, she connected erotic stimulation with her rear end. The psychology employed was to dissociate the act (absent-minded) from the feelings. In acts of adult sexuality, she dissociated as will be described below.

From early age, at least three, she practiced masturbation by stimulating clit with fingers or objects. She curled her body automatically, a position "imprinted" on her body as a child in order to conceal masturbation. Imprinting is the term used by Konrad Lorenz, Nobel Prize winner. He discovered how ducklings would forever follow any object presented to them in the early weeks of life. Although imprinting has not been proven in humans, it is an apt concept for impressions of her early experience.

A very first mental "narrative" (fantasy) that accompanied masturbation–and used again and again for many, many years–was about a situation where she was dragged into a shelter by a boy, and saw him kissing her on the mouth and touching her all over. Other boys joined and started fondling her. She spun around in the middle of a tightly knit group. Such daydreaming is a form of dissociation. Her childhood sexual fantasy is one of the few recorded in the literature.

As a very little girl playing games with her dolls, she was afforded "exquisite and incomparable sensations." She played the games in a specific and unusual way. She gathered her panties in a thick strip and wedged it into the cleft between her legs right up to her buttocks, and would sit so the fabric dug into her slightly. In that position she would take the hand of her Ken doll and let it roam over her naked Barbie. Later, she replaced the action with the panties with rubbing together the two swollen lips at the front of the cleft. Years after she had stopped playing with the dolls, she would picture herself in a situation similar to the Barbie doll, and felt she was entitled to the same caresses.

At age 11, she experienced an act by the grandfather of a girlfriend that would ordinarily be considered sexual molestation. It had very positive consequence for her psychosexual development including her first erotic emotion as such. Sitting on his lap, he brushed his hand across her budding breast. As she stayed motionless and silent, he said that when she became a woman, she would really like her "titties" stroked in this way. She turned her head against the wall as if she couldn't hear what she was being told (dissociation). However, she was aware for the first time of the stiffening of her nipples. "I was suddenly brought to the threshold of womanhood and felt a sense of pride." In connection with this event, she stated, "A child forges its power in the enigma of its future life."

Her girlfriend said he had done the same things with her. "We were pretty sure the grandfather was doing something forbidden, but the secret he gave us to share was far more valuable than some moral whose meaning was no clearer." She had processed this early sexual experience as a positive influence.

Once when she told a priest in confession about her masturbating, his reaction was "so disappointing." He just gave her a few *aves*. She felt nothing but contempt for him afterwards, and made the decision not to tell any priest about her other sexual experiences. Such disastrous experiences with the Church led her to completely abandon religion.

At age 13 or 14, she "belatedly witnessed the 'primal scene.'" He father had not slept with her mother for several years. She saw her mother with a friend when her father was away as she was kissing and arching her back in a doorway at home. Four years later the scene came to Catherine's mind when she saw her boyfriend framed in the same doorway. The mother's licentious and forbidden behavior had made an indelible impression on Catherine.

Driving down from Paris to Lyon, she had to make a stop to pee in the bushes beside the road, and a friend of her boyfriend stroked her as she squatted. It made her feel slightly embarrassed. "It was at precisely at that moment that I learned to sidestep my embarrassment by burying my head between his legs and taking his cock in my mouth."

Psychologically, she dissociated the unpleasant feelings by using a desirable sexual alternative.

Subsequently, she and boyfriend went on a car and camping trip. In the tiny tent, they had sex that allowed her to "become a woman."

The frolicking in the tent seemed to her like kid's games. They reminded her of the way she used to hide from adults by pulling a sheet up over her head succumbing to a "forbidden activity" [masturbation]. "You turn in on your intimate pleasure, pretending to ignore the fact that it might accidentally erupt in front of spectators who are not prepared for it and might even stop it." Such mental activity is normal dissociation.

Summary and conclusions about Catherine

In childhood and adolescence, Catherine related a number of sexual situations and mental states in which she utilized the normal psychological mechanism of dissociation for coping. Episodes of sibling and childhood sex play shaped some of her sexual patterns in later life. Masturbation was treasured as pleasure for her body, and persisted throughout her life. Contrary to common belief, a childhood sexual experience with an adult was positive in forming her identity. She did not consider as abnormal or traumatic any of her childhood sexual attitudes or experiences. She had no indication of sexual addiction, and she had no mental disorders. Her sexual behavior is best labeled hyper-sexuality.

Xaviera Hollander described in detail her sexual life in the book, *The Happy Hooker; My Own Story (1971)*. She stated, "From the time I lost my virginity [at age 17] I became wild about sex, and threw over my steady boyfriend in pursuit of it. I couldn't care less who I did it with, even my relatives." Her mother had advised her to keep her virginity till she was married.

Her initial falling in love was with a female classmate at age 14. "I recognized quite early that I was a natural bisexual." She attributed her "nymphomaniacal behavior" to the general South African atmosphere in which she grew up: "drunken parities creating an incestuous circle, with everyone screwing every

one else's wife or girl." She followed a life of promiscuousness with numerous boyfriends, girlfriends, and strangers. In her early twenties she had established the most famous and high-class bordello and call girl enterprise in New York City. Unlike most prostitutes, she did not engage in sex primarily for money, but did it for the sheer pleasure.

She wrote of several childhood sexual experiences and feelings. She stated that sexual expression at home was entirely natural. Since age three, she recalled seeing her father (whom she adored) walk around the house naked with an erection. "Seeing my father with a hard on was as natural as seeing my mother with a hat on." Clearly these observations of male eroticism made an impression on her.

"I have always been intrigued with beautiful breasts and even as a child I fantasized of sucking at my mother's breasts."

As a 14 year old virgin, she had a "tingling desire" to make love with her handsome brother-in-law.

At 15, she already kissed her boyfriend 'with tongue, explored his body all over, and even sucked his cock."

"In my early teens when I first heard about the facts of life from older friends, I used to wish I had a big brother so I could fuck him." In her late teens, she did "make it with some members of my family, and not by accident." At age 17, she seduced her mother's brother, her favorite uncle who adored her as a child, and as an adolescent in "a more carnal way." She thought it would be an accomplishment to make someone commit adultery that had never done it before. She turned him into "an absolute sex maniac."

When a teen babysitter, a seven-year-old boy climbed with his legs around her, somehow undid her bra, and started feeling her breast. She felt his penis becoming slightly hard. She calmed him down, and they went to lunch. This event illustrated how she showed morality and kindliness to a child with whom she allowed some freedom in natural sexual expression toward her. In early teens, she had fantasies of desire of a big brother with whom she could "fuck."

She had outstanding intellectual accomplishments at school age. She spoke seven languages fluently, and won a highest national scholastic award in high school.

Summary and comment about Xaviera

Already beginning at age three, Xaviera showed interest in her father's erections clearly evident to her in a household of natural nudity. Her mother's breasts attracted her. In her teens the erect penis and full breasts became highly attractive and erotic. She had incestuous desires at age 14, and followed through with seducing an uncle at age 17. To accomplish this intrigued her. At age 14, she had fantasies of having sex with a brother she wished for.

The data supplied showed sexual interest in father and mother at a very early age. This could represent normal interest, but could have foretold a heightened level of sexual desire in the preschool age as culminated in her intense sexual interests and behavior beginning with puberty and with losing her virginity at age 17.

She attributed her promiscuousness to the cultural atmosphere in which she grew up. One interpretation of the roots of her hyper-sexuality lies in her early childhood and teen sexual experiences. In addition, it is possible she had genetically acquired high sex drive.

Some people might call her behavior "sexual addiction." It is true that she had some of the characteristics of that so called condition, but her behavior did not interfere with her intellectual, social, or successful professional life. In no way did she have a diagnosable mental disorder. She characterized her life as one of sexual indulgence and pleasure.

CHAPTER 6

FOUR EXTREMELY SEXUAL WOMEN IN HISTORY

*N*YMPHO *AND OTHER Maniacs (*1972) contains detailed historical records of 19 women with hyper-sexuality who lived in the past four centuries. All except one were English or European, married, had been mistresses, or had multiple sexual relationships with men of fame and fortune. These included Napoleon Bonaparte and numerous royalties and writers. Only two of the case histories contain data about childhood sexuality.

Marie Duplessis

She was a mistress who inspired the great French writer, Dumas, to pen the erotic novel, *Madame Bovary.* Her grandmother had been a streetwalker and her grandfather a licentious priest. At the age of 12, she became enamored of a young farm hand where she lived on a farm, and it is said, she "left her virtue, together with her petticoat underneath a bramble bush in a hedge." At age 13, she was returned to the care of her father, a drunkard, and for a small sum of money turned her over to a wealthy, lecherous bachelor friend. He used her as he wished for a year. The operator of a restaurant near the Palais-Royal was dazzled by her beauty when she was 16. Soon, she was his mistress and provided her with luxury. Later as a teen, she supported herself as a messenger for a corset maker, and as a girl of the streets. A handsome young man, later to rise to a cabinet position in France, spotted her beauty in rough clothes and transformed her into a splendid young lady, a woman of refinement, and arbiter of taste. The story is reminiscent of the famous Greek play, Pygmalion, made into the movie, "My Fair Lady." Subsequently in order to gain her material goals, she accepted lovers in great numbers. At one time she had "a syndicate of seven ardent admirers."

She was described as a woman of incomparable charm. Franz Liszt, the famous composer and toast of Europe, fell in love with her in Paris. He confessed, "Marie was the first woman with whom I was in love." Sadly, she died of tuberculosis at the youthful age of only 23.

Nell Gwyn

In 1675, as a child she served drinks in a brothel. At this impressionable age, she was exposed to an overtly sexual environment. In teenage, she became an actress on the stage "By judiciously granting favors to the right people." (Bullough, 1964) "At the same time, she was sleeping with a succession of important men." At age 19 as a mistress of King Charles II, she lived in great luxury. When riding in a Royal Carriage and thrown insults by people on the street, she ordered the coachman to stop, put her head out the window, and shouted, "Prey good people be civil. I am a Protestant whore." At the time anti-Catholic feeling was running high. She claimed that she was "only one man's whore at a time." (Bullough, 1964) She bore the king two sons. Sadly, she died of unrecorded cause at age 21. "She died, loved if not respected by a great portion of the English people."

Victoria Woodhull

In America, she was a champion of women's' rights including suffrage, became a very successful stockbroker, prostitute, and madam of her brothel in New York City. She married at 15 years-of-age. She was the only woman in history to date to run for president of the United States. Her plank was women's rights, free love, and women's orgasm. She lost. She wrote, "I am a free lover. I have an inalienable, constitutional, and natural right to love whom I may, to love as long or short a period as I can, to change that love every day if I please. And with that right neither you nor any law you can frame will have any right to interfere." The data do not contain anything about her childhood sexuality except her young teenage marriage.

Maryellen, a woman 65 years of age in 2009 is a case of hyper-sexuality. She had a male lover fifteen years older, and tells of being turned on and feeling erotic much of the day–whenever she is alone and thinks of her lover or is in his presence. The feeling is warmth sweeping over her body and down to her pelvis that she calls a pelvic rush, a desire for touch or kiss by her lover or she to touch him, and expectation of what erotic will happen next. When he touches or kisses her any time of day or night, an excitement fills her. In bed, she is driven at least once or twice in 24 hours to touch and suck her lover's penis to point of his ejaculating in her mouth, or have intercourse.

She recalls masturbating regularly since age three. At age six, she showed first evidence of erotic attraction to boys--she took hold of a boy she liked and kissed

him. She said, "I think I shocked him." At age ten, she had strong erotic attraction to some boys her age, especially the paperboy. She had sexual attraction to a number of peer males at ages 10 to 14. At age 15, she began passionate necking including breast play, and six months later had first intercourse with a boy she liked very much. This was a relatively young age of first intercourse in the 1940s. She married at age 21, and had four children.

Her early sexual experiences are evidence of an erotic childhood and adolescence. Her eroticism and frequency of sex at age 65 is at a level that can be considered hyper-sexuality.

Conclusion

The three cases presented in more detail illustrate how positive early childhood and adolescent sexual experiences can be the precursors or cause of hyper-sexuality in female children, adults, and elderly. The other case cited showed a few positive childhood sexual events, but none negative. None of the women had traumatic or what they would consider molestation experiences. In the case of mother-son incestuous relationship, the woman had no known early sexual experience.

The data support the hypothesis that early childhood and adolescent sexual experiences can be precursors of female hyper-sexuality. More cases with detailed childhood history of hypersexual women need to be gathered.

THE LIVELY SEXUAL LIFE OF MARILYN MONROE

In a shortened life, Marilyn Monroe rose from being a rejected child raised in an orphanage and by foster parents to become a world-renowned icon of sexuality. Her fame increases today, 70 years after her death, and it continues. She achieved such incredible success by talent, beauty, working very hard, and sleeping with many of the right and most famous men in the movie business and ultimately President of the United States, J. F. Kennedy. (G. D. Jensen, 2112)

As a child, her only sexual experience was molestation and possibly rape by unknown men–all traumatic. At age 16, she dropped out of high school in L.A., and married a sailor matched by her legal guardian so that it would free her from responsibility for Marilyn. As a teen, everyone recognized her extraordinary beauty, even though she dressed plainly in hand-me-down clothes Dr. Jensen admired her in classes in Emerson Junior High School in L.A., 1939, and had a crush on her.

Between 1945 and 1947, she posed for dozens of covers of magazines. At age 23, she posed naked for a calendar. This one photo made her an instant world celebrity. It was unique and world shaking. On the cover of the first issue of *Playboy*, it made the magazine and owner Hugh Heffner famous.

She desperately wanted to become a movie actress. She slept with the influential men in the movie business to get a foothold in the movies. Agent, Jonny Hyde, 30 years older than she, discovered her, and immediately fell in love. He arranged for her first movie bit parts. He died at age 60; still wishing she would marry him. She would have stood to inherit lot of money. When people asked why she didn't marry him, she said she couldn't marry him because she didn't love him.

She slept with many men in the movie business. She was not promiscuous—she always had career reasons for having sex. After her death, a number of men claimed they had slept with her, and some had. She had affairs with many famous men in the entertainment business, including Frank Sinatra, the great singer and movie actor. She did sleep with the President of the United States, John F. Kennedy on one occasion. She was loyal to the three men she married. These included Joe DiMaggio the most famous baseball player at the time, and the very famous writer, Arthur Miller.

Sexually active and notable as she was, it is appropriate to regard her a super-sexual woman.

References

Bullough, V. L. (1964). *The History of Prostitution,* N. Y.: University Books, Inc.

Elliott, M. 1993. *Female Sexual Abuse of Children,* London: Longman Group

Hollander, X. 1972, *The Happy Hooker,* New Your: Dell Publishing

ICD-10, International Classification of Diseases, 1990. World Health Organization (WHO)

Jensen, G. D. (2012) *Marilyn; A Great Woman's Struggles.* Xlibrus Corporation

Millet, C. 2001, *The Sexual Life of Catherine M.* London: Corgi Books

www.Wikipedia, Sexual Addiction

Wallace, I. 1971, *The Nympho and other Maniacs,* New York: Pocket Books

Yates, A. 1976, *Sex Without Shame; Encouraging the Child's Early Sexual Development.* New York: Wm. Morrow and Co.

PART III

GIRLS GROWING UP TO BE HIGHLY SEXUAL

CHAPTER SEVEN SUMMARIZES a case of stepfather-child sexual rearing of daughter that eventuated in her becoming a highly sexual teenager. Many, perhaps most readers, would be uncomfortable about the possibility of parent-child sex in our culture, and would prefer to avoid the topic. That is understandable since this taboo is relatively fixed in peoples' minds, and is deeply ingrained in the mindset of society. It takes a freely open mind to venture learning more about it. To do so is to broaden knowledge. It benefits the clinician who frequently is challenged to distinguish normal healthy parent-child erotic interaction from the unhealthy, called child abuse. The reader is encouraged to read to the part on sexual abuse at the story finish. Persist! It will put positive vs. negative parent-child sexuality in perspective. The concepts presented are informative to parents and the legal system.

Chapter eight illustrates how a parent groomed a young daughter for super-sexuality. The child happens to be a beautiful, talented, movie star. In her case it did only good for her. However, it is not recommend as a pattern for childcare.

The history of intellectual growth and discovery clearly demonstrates the need for unfettered freedom, the right to think the unthinkable, discuss the unmentionable, and challenge the unchallengeable.

We value freedom of expression precisely because it provides a forum for the new, the provocative, the disturbing, and the unorthodox.

Professor Woodward, *Yale Alumni Magazine*
Nov- Dec. 2014

The history of intellectual growth and discovery clearly demonstrates the need for unfettered freedom, the right to think the unthinkable, discuss the unmentionable, and challenge the unchallengeable.

We value freedom of expression precisely because it provides a forum for the new, the provocative, the disturbing, and the unorthodox.

Professor Woodward, *Yale Alumni Magazine*
Nov- Dec. 2014

CHAPTER 7

Parents' Sexual Rearing of a Teenage Daughter Results In Her High Level of Sexuality

Note to reader

The Internet enables instant communication between persons anywhere in the world. Stephen Hawking, world famed British theoretical physicist and professor at Cambridge University, UK, wrote with assistance of his electronic communicator device, "We are all now connected by the Internet, like neurons in a giant brain." (USA Today, 12, 2, 2014; see also the Movie: *Theory of Everything*.)

The author used Internet to take medical and psychological history from a family who live in a State where the age of consent is 16. The girl in this story is 18.

In anticipation of submitting this writing, the author addressed two issues in stories of sexual interaction involving children. One is age of consent; the other is incestuous behavior and incest.

The laws of consent for sex vary greatly by country. In Japan and Argentina it is 13 years-of-age, and that Latin American country does not have a law against incest. Laws in America are not so simple as applied. The laws of sexual consent in USA are 16 or 18 years. (Federal law of consent is age 18. Age 16 is common for most of the United States).

However the legal system in America is hypocritical on how age of consent is regarded. For example, a very large federally funded scientific study of teens between ages 13 and 19 published several years ago found that the average age of experience for both sexes with either oral sex or intercourse was 15 years. A significant number of boys and girls to engaging in sex were 13 and 14 years-of-age. This means that the majority of American teens are technically breaking the laws about age of consent! The irony is, these children are never

prosecuted by the USA legal system (unless there is sexual abuse involved, and that is rare)! In other words, the American people including parents and teens ignore the law of age of consent, and engage in sex as naturally inclined. Neither any group of citizens nor does the legal systems complain. Obviously, the laws regarding consent are not working, and the current legal system is hypocritical. Unwittingly, American legal system requires, even forces children to break the law. This could cause guilt. This is damaging to mental health. It is certain that neither politicians nor legal experts working with the American criminal justice system care one iota about their mental health damage heaped on innocent children and decent law abiding American citizens. The law is not only a travesty, but is just plain confusing for childhood sex education.

It is shocking that the American legal system is so out of touch with a healthy society, and does not act sensibly or honestly. These laws are not doing well for children and parents. The same can be said about some publishers' restrictive policies about sexual material. This book gets the facts right. It will encourage parents' and the legal system to be healthy, and not continue doing harm. All need to get in step with reality.

To clarify laws about incest, there are laws against it in most countries, and all states in USA except Rhode Island. Rhode Island decriminalized incest in 1983.

The family in the case here presented in this chapter did not commit incest— the stepfather and child involved were not blood relatives. The family did not break any laws.

A preview of the case can prepare the reader. Children usually learn and experiment with sex from peers. Parents may teach sex in words, but it is unusual for them to teach sex physically by actions. This was true in this case. The mother's motive to teach was healthy. Her demonstrations to the daughter introduced her to sexual pleasuring of the stepfather, and, over nearly two years time, to mutually satisfying more extensive sex. It turned out to enjoyment and healthy growth of all, and there was no trauma or abuse. The case is analyzed scientifically for psychodynamics.

It is understood that most parents would be aghast at this family, and their erotic behavior. Probably most persons, particularly women, would immediately respond to the story with negativity, label it as "sick," and would not want to read or learn more about it. This is the cultural norm. Unfortunately it shuts down learning and growth. Few people have an open mind to healthy erotic parent-child behavior. If they allowed themselves to learn more rather than promptly judge, they could develop a more liberal mind to healthy human sexuality. They too can grow.

Because the writing in this chapter contains data about parent-child sexual interaction, a subject uncomfortable or even abhorrent to many Americans, the reader should use discretion. Children under the age of 16 should have parent permission. The story has many facts of educational merit--things children and parents would be well off to learn.

Introduction

ONE CASE IS reported in the literature of mother-son incest with positive outcome for a son, eight to 20 years-of-age (1). Only a few studies reported on cases of positive effects. (1) More such cases than expected occur, but are rarely reported.

The case reported here is of a long-term positive sexual interaction between a stepfather and older teenage stepdaughter. It is unusual, but it does happen in healthy families.

American novels have been written about stepfather and stepdaughter sexuality, and the girl is always purported to 18, the legal age of consent for several States in America. The law of consent in most of the United States is 16. In the case reported here, the girl is a resident in the State where age 16 is the legal age of consent. She is 18 years-of-age.

Child abuse is a legal concept. Father-daughter is the most common type. Mother-child abuse is the least common. One book has 15 cases of sexual abuse by mother written by the abused person. (1) Most of those cases have detailed first-person descriptions of horrendous abuse, physical, emotional and sexual began in infancy or preschool age and lasted into adolescence. Guilford Press, New York, regarded it appropriate to publish these cases in a volume on child abuse. (1)

Most all cases of parent-child sexual interaction are deemed to be sexual abuse. A review of 30 reports in the literature of parent-child sexual interaction found that most cases had negative effects, and were considered sexual abuse. Several cases were neutral and a few were positive. Miletski made a comprehensive review of the literature on mother-son incest. (2) Results showed that society believes mother-son incest is rare. "It appears that the apparent rarity of mother-son incest has more to do with society's inability to accept the idea than the taboo's strength."

The purpose of this study is to show the scientific psychodynamics in the case, to increase awareness and knowledge of father-daughter sexual interaction, and to know the difference between positive effects and sexual abuse. To know mentally positive cases in this ignored field will contribute to all professional's understanding and clinical skills. This report aims to broaden knowledge in order to better detect, possibly intervene, to educate, and to research the issues.

It is of importance to include this case in the literature in order that positive outcome cases are recognized for correct medical/psychological management, and be accurately distinguished from cases of child abuse. This story helps with that.

This account of stepfather-stepdaughter sexual interaction does not fit the definition of pornography. It cannot be considered porno. Read with discression. Children under age 16 should have parents' permission to read.

The persons in the case

The parents are university graduates, and successful professionals. The daughter was 18 years old at the start of the communication. She is physically and mentally healthy, and a bright girl. The family is Caucasian.

This family story of parent-child eroticism is authentic. About 90 e-mails were exchanged. Data was recorded in the participants' own words. This avoided bias and misinterpretation. Interspersed between the mother's e-mails, but not recorded for the story are the author's comments, answers to questions, support, and information for the mother.

The e-mail interchange was not therapy. The subjects' activities took place over the 22-month period, October 2012 to July 2014. Selected e-mails are recorded to show the style of the mother's communications. The majority of them are briefly summarized. Enough data was obtained to enable scientific analysis of psychodynamics, and to differentiate between healthy and abusive interaction.

The names of subjects and critical identifying data are changed for privacy.

Results

E-mail communications from the mother

7/10/12

Dear doctor: Good of you to hear of my story. I'd like to tell the world, but it is not something I can tell on "Oprah." My husband's name is Al, and my daughter is Ellen.

Here are our backgrounds. My husband and I have been married 10 years. He is stepfather to our daughter 18. I am 38, and my husband is 39. We live and work on the East Coast.

My girlfriend, Randy told us about chronicled reports by parents who have had positive sexual interaction with their children. Randy's personal story really touched me. It was the first time I thought such behavior wasn't dirty. I shared her story with my husband who liked it as well. It started our conversation of "Could we ever do something like that?" It was an intoxicating thought.

Our experience began with the thought of introducing my daughter to use of a vibrator. Could I just tell her how to use a vibrator, or would I really need to demonstrate on myself? Should it be just me, or should I include my husband?

I know there is no blueprint for all of this, but we would love to have tips on making this a positive experience for all of us. I think our daughter is the kind of kid that could benefit from such teaching. I would love for her to grow into a woman who is comfortable with her sexuality–more so than I was as a young woman.

How do you deal with the privacy issue? I would share with her that this is to be kept just between us. But, how do you balance that with a need to be proud of self and be honest with the world?

Randy talked with me about a couple in a similar situation. She shared with me that we need always to put our daughter first, and not give into urges to proceed faster than she can process her own wants and needs. She also said Ellen needs some control over the agenda and situation so she can make choices. Randy said, her making choices and asking for more information or demonstrations is a way to gauge her consent.

Is it appropriate to let her watch my husband and I have sex?

We have decided to sleep naked, and let her know that she can do the same if she desires.

From there, we will let her questions guide us.

I would be afraid my husband would have an erection the whole night. She might assume he is ready for sex.

7/21/12

Ellen is excited about Friday night. She really loves family night where she gets to make decisions on what we do and eat.

Last night in bed, my husband and I played out the scenario. I gave him slow hands-on stimulation while describing to Ellen what I was doing.

To our fake audience last night, I played up about how good it makes my husband feel.

I think her seeing how good it makes him feel will make her want to try doing it. Is it true that sex by my husband with our daughter could be both healthy and fun for her?

She loves giving him back rubs, and she is always happy when she elicits a moan. She loves to cuddle with her daddy.

I know it sounds like I am getting caught up in this, but really we are going to let her set the pace, and not try to entice her. We plan on letting her natural curiosity play out. Both of us are excited, but I don't want to go overboard. I want her to think it's happening organically.

I think that I will demo hand stimulating my husband.

I guess the goal would be to see if she shows interest. We think if she sees her dad in so much pleasure, she might want to try it sometime.

One quick question: If she shows interest can we expect her to be simply fascinated with it because it is new, or can we expect that she will show some level of sexual excitement? Or maybe a bit of both? Please explain.

7/30/12

Thank you Doctor for the helpful answers. Because of our excitement, we are pushing the timetable up to tonight.

We plan on lounging in bed, watch her movies, and eating pizza. We will explain that we sleep naked, and she can also if she wants.

I trust you, and I trust Randy after all the time I spent chatting with her.

Last night was beautiful. In demo, I stimulated my husband. Ellen was fascinated, and asked questions. I finished him.

Quick note: When I was touching him, he let out a moan that sounded so pleasurable. She asked, "Did that feel good?" All the while knowing what pleasure he had.

This morning, we talked about privacy.

8/12/12

We had a marvelous weekend together as a family. We had lots of loving family fun, in and out of bed.

It really makes us question why anyone would think this is wrong?

She imitated me in stimulating my husband. I really think she enjoyed playing with him. She acted sultry, something I had never seen before.

The next night, Friday, we watched TV in bed, and again Al got naked, and ready for bed.

Wide eyed, she commented to me that he was hard again.

I asked her, "What do we do about it? She laughed and said, "Ask Dad."

A few minutes later in bed, I moved so that my husband was in the middle, and I started to rub him lightly.

Ellen was watching, and asked if we were going to do the same thing tonight. I said yes, and asked if she wanted to do it again. She said, "yes."

She seemed to "jump" back in when my husband showed signs close to climax.

Finally, I asked her if she wanted to finish him, and she said yes.

Al was pretty close to the edge. When he spurted up like a fountain, she was both enthralled and amazed. Again, she learned something. She was pretty proud of herself.

After we cleaned him up, we talked about it, and she talked about wanting to stimulate him from start to finish next time. My husband and I said she could. He

said he would like it from her. The comments he makes to her obviously excite her.

Seeing all this, I was amazingly horny, and we had a demo session of my husband performing on me.

I came pretty quickly. Watching this, she acted mature and interested.

When I finished, she said "wow" a lot. We talked about the taste and smell of women, and the need to be clean. (She was the one asking questions)

My husband took the next step by telling her that if interested, they could try the same thing. She was quiet for a bit, and then said that she wasn't sure.

We assured her that it was completely up to her. Ellen finally did ask her dad to do like he did with me. She asked different questions, and we talked more.

The forgoing direct conversations are sufficient to give the reader indications of the manner in which the mother and stepfather began teaching sexuality. Months of interaction that followed are summarized. Then, the direct communications are resumed.

The parents introduced Ellen to sexual interaction. Soon, she became orgasmic with the stimulation. Over a period of weeks, she became hooked on it. She asked him to promise never to stop doing it. They came to engage in this sexuality on a regular basis. Usually, Ellen was the one who initiated it. She had no problem being naked. Sometimes the mom was present to observe, and other times they were alone. Always, they went at a pace set by Ellen.

9/10/12

As far as sleeping arrangements go, Ellen is between us. We are all usually naked although Ellen sometimes wears a nightshirt.

We saw a change in Ellen when she is playing with us. Like I said before, she can be downright sultry.

Ellen had seen me demo sex on my husband. I told her that it on him was something that just I do for him. I think she is content just touching him. If she shows any desire to perform any more intense sex on him, we will revisit the matter.

Curiosity did get the best of Ellen during my demo of sex on my husband tonight. She took the initiative, and imitated me. She didn't do it for long, maybe less than a minute, and she told him to wait and not to climax.

He said it was about the best, and couldn't believe how it made him feel.

She finished him with her hands only. He spurted sperm as usual. She is still pretty proud when that happens.

9/12/12

Can girls her age get horny? I know she looks forward to it, and gets excited, but is it horny, or is that something that comes with puberty and the hormones? [The Doctor e-mailed answered her questions with explanations of normal sexual development.]

As far as our sexual activities go, I demoed on my husband till he came. Ellen was amazed, and as turned on as I've seen her.

I think that she is intrigued by the fact that semen is edible. We talked about how eating and drinking sweet things can make semen more palatable. We tested it once with him drinking pineapple juice, and the results were amazing. It was actually sweet.

We joke that we will change his diet in order to get her to enjoy it.

One of Ellen's biggest changes has been that she is more verbal when receiving sex. She will let him know what feels good and what she likes. She says things like, "more, more, yeah just like that, I want it. God it feels good!" It looks like she has had some mind blowing orgasms that put her right to sleep. Ha-ha, just like my husband! My husband is thrilled beyond belief that he gets to experience ANY of this.

We have talked about intercourse, and plan on demoing it more. That might be a line we will not cross with her.

9/29/12

Doctor, we missed you last week. We just got back today from a small vacation. We are deliriously happy with how things have panned out for our family.

Ellen has had voracious appetite for knowledge and pleasure both giving and receiving.

She asked me "What else do you and daddy do?" I have run out of pleasures to describe.

Since I last e-mailed, we have demoed intercourse. Ellen was on the bed with us, and was interested. She asked if it felt good for my husband even though I had a baby. We laughed a bit at that question, and explained that after delivery the vagina gets tight again.

And, yes indeed, in answer to your question, my husband enjoys making love with me.

10/1/12

You asked about the vibrator. There is nothing to say about it. Although the idea of that is how this all started, we haven't bothered to introduce her to it.

Besides, she pleasures herself by self-touch about every day after school. She says it relaxes her. She is very positive about it. I reinforce her by telling her, "good going." She always smiles at my positive comments.

I'm there in our bed with them most of the time, but occasionally when they are alone, they "play."

She sleeps with us about 3 or 4 times a week now. Nudity is random.

She and my husband are definitely closer, in and out of bed. Like I said, she has always been a cuddly kid. She seems more self-confident.

By sultry, I meant that her personality changes slightly when she is tending to my husband. I can see that she knows that she is in control, and can bring him pleasure.

I am comfortable with her there watching us making love.

So, do you suggest drawing the line at intercourse? Given her age, is it ever healthy?

Regarding her peers, Ellen has both boy and girl friends, and they visit at their homes. She excels at school, is into sports (soccer), and extracurricular activities. She is tall, stately, and slim.

We have been progressing with Ellen's education--lots to talk about. She has shown some signs of possession of my husband. Sometimes she wants him all to herself. At other times, she is fine with all three of us together. Also, she thinks that she has to be at ALL of my husband's and my love making sessions. Sometimes, I feel that we have to sneak behind her back.

She and I still have a great relationship, but I get the feeling that she wants to be the Alpha female. By that I mean she wants to be top woman in the pecking order. Lol. With kindness, I'll make sure she knows her place.

10/2/12

I owe you an update. Ellen has grown so much recently as we have grown as family. We have achieved a nice balance of her needs, and how that fits into my husband's and my relationship.

11/13/12

I wanted to reach out, and give you an update. This is it, and my husband approves. First off, all is well with us--actually, better than good. I'm pregnant! We are all super excited, Ellen included. We knew for a while, but I didn't mention it because I worried that that could compromise our anonymity. We are due in March.

I hope that it doesn't change the family dynamic that has been so perfect for the past couple of months.

My husband and I have struck a great balance with Ellen's newfound "hobby." Ha-ha, I kid. But seriously, it is amazing how mature this has made her.

My husband has made their relationship all about Ellen in that she is receiving most of the pleasure, and he is on the receiving end when Ellen feels like it. That comes and goes.

1/5/13

Here is a long overdue update. In the past few weeks, Ellen has asked to be present at our lovemaking including intercourse. We allowed it most of the times. She is fascinated, and asks lots of questions like how often we do it, how it feels to each of us, and why we don't use a condom like she learned in sex Ed class at school. We explain all; it's almost like a class.

Although things are going well, Ellen is pushing boundaries. She is eager for intercourse, but we are not interested in taking that route with her as yet. She just isn't ready for that next step. But, it is getting increasingly hard making that point with her.

We just don't want her going too fast. She needs to be satisfied with what we are doing now.

Part of the fun is watching her learn. Things we take for granted, she has to learn. For example, she assumed that when my husband has orgasms, he is pushing his cum out, making it squirt like urine. She had made a comment about him "not pushing hard" when he had a less than spectacular orgasm. We explained that when a man has orgasm, he is just along for the ride, and the orgasm happens almost involuntarily.

I love hearing her ask questions like that.

1/10/13

Life has got a lot simpler and less busy now that the holidays are over.

One evening, my husband and Ellen were "playing" sexually. Again, she asked about intercourse. My husband told her that that his member was too big, and she wasn't big enough for it.

She said quickly. "Well, my vibrator fits, and your thing isn't THAT much bigger." He was surprised that she had even tried inserting the vibrator. Well, when he heard that, he said, "Show me." She retrieved the vibrator, and showed him. Although it is almost an inch wide, to our amazement it slipped right in. Even she said there was never any discomfort whenever she used the vibrator internally.

It is a battery-powered vibrator that I gave her. She said she uses it masturbating. It is hers now. I never used it. It was a cheap one that was a

joke-gift a few years ago. It is fairly thin. It is my understanding that she sometimes masturbates with it after school.

As far as sex with my husband goes, we didn't want to set an expectation for her to do everything she sees us doing. Ellen continues to be curious about intercourse, but we want to take it slow, and take more time before possibly encouraging her taking that step.

1/15/13

In answer to your question about frequency of sex, it is almost every day. Of course, she likes it! Who wouldn't!

On that note, we have been careful with definitions of things. We don't want her vocabulary to betray her so we have been using "play" for the sexual activity, although we also call it "making love." Defining orgasms has been harder. She knows the word "orgasm," as well as the meanings of "almost there" and "close to it."

Neither of us is jealous. She gives us time for our own lovemaking, and I give them the room they need.

She doesn't ask for demonstrations anymore, but she has sometimes watched us when we make love.

1/20/13

I don't know if I could say that she has become more erotic because she has been super sultry since all this started. She has become more confident in her lovemaking. I think she knows a lot more, knows what she is doing, and what to expect. She is a great communicator during sex. She isn't afraid to tell my husband what she wants and likes.

In answer to your questions, yes, when co-sleeping we are all usually naked. There are no rules. Like I said, she likes to cuddle. When naked in bed, she cuddles with my husband. She does curl up with me sometimes when watching TV or reading.

My husband and I also have had more sex since the new situation. Even with the extra demand on him, we are having significantly more sex now. And even with my pregnancy!

Ellen is happy with the vibrator. Although she has put it inside her, she said that is not the way she masturbates. She masturbates by pressing it on along her clit and slit.

My husband and I have talked about having a vasectomy. He feels that when intercourse happens, it would make it much simpler for him, and safer. I also like the idea because I don't plan any more children. He has an appointment with the doctor next week to find out all about it.

2/4/13

Ellen is super excited about the baby due next month. She is curious how he will be involved with all of us. We may need some guidance from you, Doctor, on that

2/10/13

My husband and Ellen went away on his business trip. He had events in the same hotel they were staying at. She was able to stay in the room during the time he was out, and still be connected by cell phone. I was afraid that she was going to be bored, but she loved the appearance of independence.

He said that Ellen "loooooooved" being alone with him. They had plenty of snuggling. He said, he felt like they were lovebirds on honeymoon.

There is one story of their interaction when she and my husband were away together.

Well, when she was pleasuring him, his hips involuntarily moved up and down. She told him that he didn't have to do that, and that he could stop moving his hips. He explained that everyone's hips have a mind of their own when it comes to sex, and will just move on their own.

Yes, my husband praises me as well, and I believe the nature of their relationship makes ours more exciting. I don't think that I'm losing him to her. I know that I am loved. In fact, this whole experience has made us closer. We talk more now. There is trust. And, we turn each other on. I don't mind that he and Ellen have the special relationship. It has brought all of us closer.

She isn't addicted to sex; she just loves it. I think she loves the intimacy as much as the orgasms. Ellen loves him as a father, and not as romantic love.

2/24/13

Last week was school vacation. We were away for just a few days, and got back before the weekend. Our family loves the intimacy of it all, like it is in a special grown up club.

I asked my husband for details about being away together alone with Ellen. He said that they slept naked, but spent much of the time clothed.

She is definitely broadening her boundaries with sex and initiating it more. I've seen her rub him through his pants while cuddling and watching TV in the living room next to the kitchen.

Yes, their open mouth kissing is new.

2/24/13

He said their time away lent itself to giving each other pleasure. Including an hour-long oral session on her. I don't think that I was missed. Lol.

2/25/13

If others only could only understand this lifestyle for families! It's the stigma that society places on these situations that are harmful.

Amazingly, I am jealous and envious of his relationship with Ellen. I can't believe how lucky I am. Although my husband gets to experience the pleasure directly, I am blessed to be able witness it, and see how much joy they bring to each other.

I melt when I see Ellen on the verge of orgasm. Such an amazing expression on her face! Seeing them, I realize that they are really connected at the heart. Sorry to get so poetic.

5/3/13

It's a turn on for me to see my husband and Ellen together sexually. I think the whole situation has supercharged everyone's libido.

3/7/13

Last night, Ellen was tired, and not feeling well so went to bed early. This gave my husband and I time to be together without her. It was nice for just the two of us.

Although the three of us have a heightened libido, it doesn't show around our extended family, friends or coworkers. In public, we act as an ordinary natural friendly family.

I have seen them have lip-to-lip kisses. I think, he must have taught her how. Or could it be natural inspiration in the heat of passion? I remember it was that way for me as a virgin teen. I couldn't get over it, wanted it all the time, and got it with my boyfriend. My libido skyrocketed. It was so good beyond description. I can feel it even now.

3/8/13

My fantasies are born from jealousy. I see my husband and E interact, but I can't experience it like he does.

3/9/13

Well, Al didn't get the "semen all clear" just yet. The technician commented that he couldn't understand the immediate need to prematurely check the active sperm count with a wife who is pregnant! Ha-ha. Let it be a mystery for him. Al will go back in a few weeks for one last check.

Last night was TV-in-bed Friday night. Well, the TV didn't last that long.

3/9/13

Yes, last night everyone was naked, and all of us slept together. I think the consensus was, "wow, that was fun!"

After he and I made love, the three of us talked about his sperm viability test. He told her that if she wanted to try to continue trying to lower the count, she should feel free.

When Al and I had intercourse, I was lying on my side, and he entered form the rear, the position I particularly crave.

After we finished, Ellen commented that my husband was moving fast. I knew she was referring to our thrusting. :) I'm sure that there will be a future lesson on making love. And yes, the night was pretty hot.

3/10/13

Ellen's comment about him moving fast was about when he was in me.

3/10/13

In answer to your question, no, with Ellen we don't use the word fuck***. My husband has uttered it while receiving oral from her. He didn't do it on purpose, but it slipped out in a moment of ecstasy. He explained why he said it. She understood.

3/11/13

I saw kissing during their lovemaking, but it wasn't aggressive kissing; just loving lip-to-lip contact. Also, "It makes one kinda wish..."

3/11/13

I talked about Ellen's wetness when with my husband. He said that she is usually wet inside when they have sex play.

Yes, I am in the room with them quite often during their sexual interaction, but he is the one who has the real front row seat. I would love to be a fly on the wall, and see how they interact without me there.

3/12/13

Here's a little about Ellen's appearance. She has brown hair down past her shoulders, slender body, olive skin, long legs, and is tall. A very pretty girl, she is. She likes her body, and we are very proud parents.

3/13/13

Just saw your question, Doctor: Am I comfortable with Ellen watching my husband and me making love?" Yes, I am comfortable with her being there watching us.

3/19/13

Yes, Ellen and her dad have always been close, but are even closer now. She was always his little buddy. She always liked to snuggle and cuddle, but more so now, and it's stronger. In bed, she likes clinging to him.

4/4/13

We had to have a talk with Ellen this past week. She has become a little possessive with my husband. I think she gets it now, but I can see this happening again.

With the baby nursing, and my lack of sleep, I have not been my normal horny self. Ellen benefits because it allows more opportunity for her to be with her dad.

This week, I wanted some alone time together with Al, but Ellen wanted to sleep in our bed with us. Not to be allowed this one time, she was disappointed, and got pouty.

4/5/13

Yes, I can see how her jealousy could cause a chuckle, but we weren't laughing when it happened. It ruined our time together, but then again, we are the ones that opened Pandora's box.

I really think that Ellen gets it, and understands that we need time alone without her. But, when it happens, she doesn't recognize the situation as

reasonable. All she knows is that she is being left out. We will have to work with her on that.

Although she was better the next day, I can see it happening again. After all, I don't know how rational a horny 18 year-old kid can be.

5/5/13

We're both great with including her in our everyday life. We focus on her after school sports activities, and include her in everything we all do like shopping, trips, and fun things.

We are only getting resistance to her sharing Al in regard to bedroom activity.

5/8/13

Friday was date night for my husband and me. Ellen slept at a friend's house. It was nice just being with friends. I'm flattered that they like to run hands over my big belly, and it feels good when they touch it. With the baby coming, our lives are about to get busy.

We were inspired Saturday afternoon when Ellen got back home from her over night with a girlfriend. We talked with her, and Al explained that if she wanted to tease him it's OK.

After 10 minutes of his caring, she was so turned on basically, she begged him to let her climax. And, he let her. I think she is more about an instant gratification than a slow build up.

I learned that she does better with encouragement than direction. She views me telling her how to do something as a critique, so instead I praise her when she does the right things. For her, my husband on the other hand can do no wrong. She takes his comments, good and bad, to heart.

3/19/13

I am tempted to organize an extended session for both of them tonight.

3/19/13

Can't wait for my body to get back in shape to enjoy the two of them with me in a participatory role. I agree with Al that he is one lucky guy--you might say, a living dream.

Ellen knows the power that she has over him, but I think she realizes that he holds power, as well.

3/24/13

Well, I have perfected the technique of giving long-time oral sex to Al. Ellen is also getting better at it. This bodes well for my husband.

Yes, Ellen can have more than one orgasm with a rest in between anywhere from five minutes to an hour. It depends on her level of horniness that is actually near constant 24/7 every day of the week.

3/28/13

Well, intercourse hasn't happened yet. That is why I haven't brought it up. My husband doesn't want to hurt her, so he doesn't push for it. Ellen loves so much what they do that I think she doesn't mind waiting a little longer. I'm certain it will happen in due time. She says she can't wait. Meanwhile, she can't get enough sex always with love from her dad

4/14/13

I thought Ellen might be a little jealous because all the focus has been on the baby.

Tonight was movie night in bed. The movie ended, and she is currently giving my husband pretty amazing touching. So slow and thoughtful! She has him in heaven. 30 minutes ago, he announced that he was moments away from climax. She seems to be able to go on forever. Poor guy! Lol. But, she loves it. It's her favorite thing. She is getting a little sex crazed. Lucky girl!

He is threatening to tease her as well. She doesn't seem concerned. This is quite a show I have front row tickets to.

Ellen finally put him out of misery. Lol.

He returned the favor by teasing her for close to 40 minutes. I was half dosing through it, but I heard her desperate voice begging to let her . . . I think she just wanted to get off; she was teasing him. There were times he would pull away, and she was frustrated enough to try and push herself over the edge.

4/15/13

Regarding masturbation, I don't know about her "always" having orgasm.. Although I have witnessed Ellen having powerful orgasms, I do not think that they are yet on par with mine. Ha-ha.

4/15/13

Ellen has a jump on me by years. By the time she is in latest teens, she will catch up to me. I know that will be a blast. I wonder how many boyfriends she will take? Any one could be so lucky. I will advise her when the time comes.

4/30/13

No, I wouldn't say that Ellen is sex addicted. I remember saying that she isn't addicted to sex, but she does love it. In my message, I may have meant that once they start intercourse, she would like it too much. Right now, she sex craved for everything he does to her. My husband gives to her seemly all she can take, but she still wants more of the same. At her age and desire, I say it's good to be greedy. We do praise her for everything she does.

5/12/13

He does service her plenty, but she gets jealous when seeing Al and I having sex without her chance to participate.
Recently, she has been cooperative in giving us our time alone. I am amazed at her maturity.

5/14/13

With regard to the question of how often she masturbates to orgasm now, it really depends on her mood. Counting orgasms with Al, she has a total of at least 10 times a week.

5/16/13

Ellen knows that I am e-mailing a medical doctor who is advising us.
Another business trip with Al is in her future. I don't mind giving them the alone- time. They are so much closer now than where they were a year ago. Not to say that they weren't close. They are just way closer now.

12/12/13

I noticed that Ellen acts a bit sexy when her step-uncle visits. He is Al's 28 year-old-brother. E asked me if I would invite him to come when my husband and I are out, "so we could be alone." Without knowing more, I understood her desire. I set it up by asking him to be with E when we would be away overnight. I told him in advance not be surprised if she asks him to be intimate like taking

him to bed. I said, "She is old enough to give consent." He said that he thought he could handle it.

The next day, she told me about their visit. Right off, she asked him to go to bed and have sex. He was a bit shy, but they did have it. They slept in her bed. In the morning he awakened to see her self-pleasuring. Then, he went home. They had a wonderful time.

I gave her my blessings. This same morning, she was on the phone with him for about an hour, and afterward was giddy like a teen with a crush.

This was the first time Ellen had talked sex on the phone. She has reached the stage of development that she communicates directly what kind of sex she wants to do with a partner, and what she wants done to her.

1/20/14

We were to be away overnight again, and to Ellen's delight, I asked Al's brother to again stay with E. This time without hesitation, he was eager. Ellen reported they repeated the same intimacy with more pleasure than the first time. I'm not encouraging her to continue their visits, but have decided to go along with her expressed wishes.

He is not only handsome, but a very sexy, gentle, and a kind young man. We have always gotten along well. Al is accepting and even pleased with Ellen's relationship with the uncle--he said so. Al's approval made Ellen feel good. Every child wants their parents' recognition and praise, you know.

Summary of the next 6 months

Several months ago, Ellen enticed her stepfather to introduce her to intercourse. It went very tenderly and easily, and became a regular part of their lovemaking. She initiated lovemaking about 50 percent of the times. She is always orgasmic, and multiply orgasmic at times. I often observed them.

Author's discussion of the case

This girl did not have any sexual experiences or direct parental teaching of sexuality prior to the mother's program of eroticism training. Stepparent-stepchild sexual behavior was new for her at age 18.

The girl's mother presented information to analyze psychodynamics. The mother began the training of daughter with motivation to help her become more comfortable with sexuality as an adult in contrast to her relatively restricted education growing up. Her feeling of pleasure seeing daughter learning and having sex with stepfather, her feeling proud of daughter's sexual expressions with him, and her pleasure literally observing daughter's sexual interaction

could mean not only achievement of her goals of being a good parent, but also identification with daughter to have satisfactions and pleasures she did not have. These are things every healthy mother wants for her child.

The mother was openly accepting of Ellen's talk about sex. This represents the family's unusual degree of freedom verbally expressing their sexuality, and especially for Ellen at age 18.

In adolescent phase of development, Ellen is already off the charts for ordinary girls her age. Her sexual system can be called hyper-erotic and hypersexual, or simply normal highly sexual! Being both things would be good for a girl or mature woman of any age. It bodes well for her when attaining full sexual maturity in youth and young adulthood. She would never brag to friends, as is common among teenagers. She has learned to be discreet.

With regard to masturbation, she does it ever day with fingers, and always comes rather quickly. Total orgasms per month for her are around 210. Her "cup runneth over." She never feels unfulfilled sexually. She feels horny much of the day. Adult women can be envious. Few women of any age attain her frequency level of complete sexual outlet. She never feels guilt or shame. That spells well for mental and physical health. She is special! And, she is fortunate to have such healthy sexually liberal parents.

Parents love their children, and want to be and do the best for them. The area of childhood sexuality is difficult for most parents, or the single parent. Inhibition or negativity often prevails. With the issue of incest, social custom and the "taboo" conflicts both behavior and emotions.

This family has shown how an adolescent daughter expressed eroticism, and how the parents began and proceeded slowly in steps leading to extensive sexual expression. Long-term follow-up would ascertain consequences for the child's eventual sexual and mental health. Two years after beginning sexual teaching by Mother, the girl was physically and mentally healthy, and had attained a wide range and high frequency of real sexual experiences.

All family members were highly pleased with the process and results of family sexuality. The interviewer monitored the family behavior as reported by mother to insure it was health promoting, and not sexual abuse.

The mother's motivation was to initiate and pursue sexual teaching. She wished her daughter to become more mature sexuality than she had been growing up.

Her method of sexual training and interaction included:

- open discussion of language to be used about sexuality
- direct discussion of social custom about sexual interaction in their family context
- verbal and non-verbal instruction

- allowed child to openly observe husband-wife's sexuality (modeling)
- demonstration of sexual interaction patterns as appropriate, and at the child's pace
- allowed child to take the lead in imitating mother
- care to avoid pressure or overwhelming influence (avoiding certain sexuality "too soon")
- allowed child to initiate sexual interactive behavior
- gave child permission to self-pleasure
- accepted child's curiosity
- discussed with husband to reach mutual agreement on sexual actions and teaching
- husband in concert with wife in plans and actions for teaching
- encouraged the child to ask questions, and act as she felt comfortable
- mother's occasional observation and monitoring child-stepfather sexual interaction
- support and positive reinforcement for all aspects of behavior
- praised the child's successes and affection of parents
- all sexuality done within the context of family solidarity and loving care

Summary of this family's sequential steps teaching Ellen sexuality:

- Mother demonstrated to daughter masturbation of husband
- By self, daughter performed sexual stimulation of stepfather up to ejaculation
- Husband demonstrated giving wife oral sex
- At daughter's request, stepfather gave her sexual stimulation to extent of orgasm
- Daughter took to giving sex to stepfather to point of ejaculation
- Family was discrete about their sexual activity
- They created a family bed
- All slept in family bed several times a week
- Naked in bed, daughter cuddled stepfather
- Daughter showed increased interest in parents' intercourse, and wanted to observe more of their lovemaking; parents allowed it
- Daughter's communication about sex with mom and dad expanded
- Daughter asked stepfather to give her intercourse; he accepted the invitation, and all members of family were happy with the results
- Daughter used dildo vibrator on pubis, and inserted it into vagina to learn size of vagina
- Family settled down to a satisfying and rewarding regular pattern of sexual interaction.
- Family felt more loving, content, and sexually fulfilled

o without a clear acceptance and understanding by the child at all times
o the perpetrator acts for own emotional and/or sexual gratification
o secretly persuading a child to engage in sex or photography for pornography
o use of alcohol or drugs
o holding the child in captivity
o impregnating the child
o passing on sexually transmitted infection

One or more of the above elements are present in **all** cases of abuse. In legal terminology there is the perpetrator and the victim. In a high percentage of such cases consequent trauma and damage to mental health occurs.

Oprah Winfrey said to Barbara Walters (Barbara Waters *CBS special on the 10 most influential persons in 2014*, December 2014) that she was 42 years old when she finally realized how those men who had molested her in childhood had *manipulated* her. She was impregnated by one and delivered a baby at age 15. She had to withstand her father's accusing her of shame for it. The infant died. On worldwide TV network viewed by countless millions of people, she told of it bravely and freely. In so doing, she shows how she has overcome the childhood trauma of horrendous sexual abuse. On her own TV show, she has featured the problem of sexual abuse several times. These are a public service.

The stepfather's sexual and loving interaction in Ellen's case was healthy, and growth promoting. It promoted stronger family bonds and loving. It appeared to further the girl's happiness and maturity.

What were the mindsets of mother and father? Both presented sufficient data to analyze psychodynamics. The mother began the training of daughter with motivation to help her become more comfortable with sexuality as an adult in contrast to her relatively restricted education growing up. Her feeling of pleasure seeing daughter learning and having sex with the stepfather, her feeling proud of daughter's sexual expressions with him, and her pleasure literately observing daughter's sexual interaction could mean not only achievement of her goals of being a good parent, but also identification with daughter to have satisfactions and pleasures she did not have when a young woman. These are things every healthy mother wants for her child. The mother never had any direct sexual interaction with her as she demonstrated some sexual acts and explained sex. This did not constitute incest--there was never mother-daughter incest.

With open discussion, all family members overcame societies attitude about the taboo of parent-child sexual interaction. They were discrete, and completely honest with each other. This built family cohesion, again mentally healthy. The increased pleasure in wife-husband sex life, an offshoot of the family sexual behavior, could have added motivation to enlarge on and encourage the stepfather's sexual interaction with the daughter. None of the participants had guilt or shame about their choices, a factor of sound mental health.

This case is unique in the literature in that both parents together were involved in teaching sexual behavior.

Why did the father participate? He felt comfortable in concert with his wife's sexual training program of training in sex and intercourse. It was not only pleasurable to him, but gave him the feeling he was being a loving father. It can be inferred that his pleasures were like his daughter's. He did not exploit her. All healthy fathers' actions and motivations are of such type. The stepfather's sexual acts with the girl did not constitute incest according to the technical and legal definitions of the word.

The stepfather felt comfortable in concert with his wife's sexual training program, and with subsequent father-daughter sex and intercourse. It was not only pleasurable to him, but gave him the feeling he was being a loving father. It can be inferred that his pleasures were like his daughter's. He did not exploit her. All healthy fathers' actions and motivations are of such type.

The e-mail doctor-parent interchange was not therapy. If a therapist were to encounter such a situation as this case in a clinical setting, they could elect to offer therapy or counseling. If the parent accepted therapy, it would be characterized as giving important facts, and explaining consequences of parent-child sexual interaction. Information about non-abusive behavior would be spelled out, and abuse would be warned against. Protection of the child's mental health is paramount.

Summary of the case

This case is one in which the stepdaughter is age of sexual consent, 18 years-of age. Details of the case are presented to document the process and psychodynamics of developing healthy parent-child sexual interaction patterns in this single case. It shows how the sexual interaction between stepfather and stepchild was healthy and growth promoting to the child. Since stepfather and child were not were not blood relatives, technically, incest was not an issue. The stepfather's sexual acts with the girl did not constitute incest according to the technical and legal definitions of the word. Nevertheless, in our culture, most people would consider some of the sexual interaction a moral issue, or immoral.

In this case, the daughter's eroticism blossomed, and the parents' sexuality also benefited. They were joyous in all interaction. Readers will be pleasantly surprised if they read completely with an open mind. There was never any child abuse. Characteristics of healthy sexual interaction are contrasted with that of child sexual abuse. The intent of the report is education. Presented are facts and analysis.

Although this case of stepparent-child sexuality was legal, and turned out to be emotionally healthy for the entire family, be aware that this writing does not recommend sexual interactive behavior of parents and child.

References

1. Elliott, M. (Ed.) (1994). *Female sexual abuse of children*, New London: The Guilford Press (pp. 113-197)
2. Miletski, H. (2005). *Mother-son Incest: the Unthinkable Taboo.* VT: Safer Society Press

CHAPTER 8

CHILDHOOD SEXUALIZATION OF A FAMOUS MOVIE STAR, NATALIE WOOD

THE HISTORY OF the beautiful very successful Hollywood movie star, Natalie Wood has many similarities to the sexual up bring of Ellen (Chapter 7).

Natalie became a star of movies at age six. (1) "Many ex-employees on the 20th Century-Fox studio lot said she was already making eyes at older men when she was just 10 years old." A publicist who knew Natalie well, said, "She seemed for too mature for her age." Her first sexual encounter was at age 14. Her mother arranged it with Nick Adams, then 23, a close friend of the family. Adams said that the matchmaking mother explained to him, "She's going to be doing it anyway, and I'd rather it be with you. I know I can trust you." He was reportedly not "her lover for long." "Soon there were a lot of guys a lot older than she was, or even me, taking her out," said the director of the classic movie, **Rebel Without a Cause**, in his forties at the time. The public read about her making rounds at nightspots with actor Raymond Burr, who at age 39 was old enough to be her father.

It is clear that Natalie's mother encouraged her daughter's early sexuality (being sultry by making eyes at adult men when she was 10 years old), and by giving permission for sex, and setting up her first intercourse at age 14. This compares with Ellen's mother teaching oral sex that led to intercourse at age 18.

When being sexual, Ellen was above the legal age of consent in her native country. When Natalie was sexual, she was under the legal age of consent in America. She was sexually active in her teens, as are most normal adolescents in America. An important point to note is the role the two mothers played in

promoting their child's active sexuality. In each case, they acted to build good mental health. No child abuse ever happened.

Reference

1. Austin, J. (1990). *Hollywood's Unsolved Mysteries*, New York: Shapolsky Publishers

www.ingramcontent.com/pod-product-compliance
Lightning Source LLC
Chambersburg PA
CBHW050419290526
45786CB00003B/1325